THE PROSTATE CANCER ESSENTIALS FOR SURVIVAL SERIES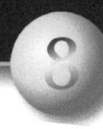

CONQUERING PROSTATE CANCER WITH DART AND BRACHYTHERAPY

MICHAEL J. DATTOLI, MD

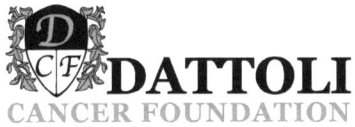

SARASOTA, FLORIDA

Prostate Cancer Essentials for Survival Series: Conquering Prostate Cancer with DART and Brachytherapy

Copyright © 2022–2026 by Michael J. Dattoli

All rights reserved. No part of this work may be reproduced or transmitted in any form or by any means, electronic or mechanical, including photocopying or recording, or by any information storage or retrieval system, except as may be expressly permitted by the 1976 Copyright Act or in writing by the publisher.

ISBN-10: 1-7212556-7-2
ISBN-13: 978-1-7212556-7-2

Published by the Dattoli Cancer Foundation, Sarasota, FL

Book design and composition by Daniel van Loon, Batavia, IL
Book edits and revisions by Design Corps, Colorado Springs, CO

MEDICAL DISCLAIMER

This book is intended as a supplement but not as a substitute for the medical advice of a physician. It is imperative that you consult a qualified healthcare professional with regard to all matters relating to your health and particular situation. Neither the publisher nor the authors bear responsibility for any consequences due to the reader's decision to use any particular treatment, medication, dietary supplement or other healthcare practices discussed in this book.

DEDICATION

This booklet is dedicated to all those whose lives have been touched by prostate cancer, and to the patients and their families whom we are privileged to serve and educate as cancer care providers.

ACKNOWLEDGMENTS

We are deeply grateful to a number of people who have contributed to this booklet. Our thanks to Greg Lawrence, for his editorial efforts and to Ginya Carnahan, Chris Wells, Joney Fay, and Amber Kawlewski at the Dattoli Cancer Center & Brachytherapy Research Institute for their ongoing assistance. We also want to thank Jennifer Cash ARNP, MS, for her long association and many contributions to the Dattoli Cancer Foundation and this booklet series.

    We deeply appreciate all of those wonderful patients and family members who have contacted the Dattoli Cancer Foundation for counseling and guidance and in turn have given us their support and encouragement. It is your spirit and commitment in confronting this disease that inspires us all.

CONTENTS

INTRODUCTION

The Essential Tools for Fighting Prostate Cancer 9

OVERVIEW—IMRT WITH DART, AND BRACHYTHERAPY

What is Radiation and How Does It Work? 12
What is External Beam Radiation Therapy? 13
What are the Risks of Side Effects with External Radiation? 14
What is 3D-Conformal Radiation Therapy? 15
What is Intensity Modulated Radiation Therapy? 16
How is IMRT Planned and Performed? 16
What is Dynamic Adaptive Radiotherapy (DART)? 17
What are the 4D IG-IMRT Analysis Tools for Image Guidance to Achieve DART? 20
How does IMRT Compare to 3D-CRT? 22
Which Patients are Eligible for External Radiation Therapy? 23
What is Brachytherapy? 24
Dr. Dattoli on the Choice of Brachytherapy Isotopes 26
Dr. Dattoli on Treating Metastatic Disease with DART 31
What is High Dose Rate (HDR) Brachytherapy? 36
How are Permanent Seed Implants Planned and Performed? 37
Which Patients are Eligible for Brachytherapy? 41
What are the Most Common Myths About Brachytherapy? 43
When is Hormonal Therapy used in Conjunction with Seeding and External Radiation? ... 46
What is Neoadjuvant Hormonal Therapy? 46
What are the Possible Side Effects of Seed Implantation? 47
What is the Risk of Erectile Dysfunction After Seed Implantation? 49
How Do Seed Implants Affect Sexual Activity? 50
What Precautions Should Patients Exercise after the Implant Procedure? 51
How are Implants Modified for Patients with Prior TURPs? 51
What are the Advantages of Palladium-103 Over Iodine-125? 52
What are the Advantages of Combining Seed Implants with External Radiation Therapy? ... 52
Why Should Seed Implants Be Done After External Radiation? 53

What are the Results of the Dattoli Combined Radiotherapy Protocol? 54

What is a PSA Bounce? 56

*What Are RapidArc™, Volumetric Modulated Arc Therapy (VMAT),
And The TrueBeam™ System?* 56

What Is The Calypso® 4D Localization Tracking System? 59

What Is TomoTherapy®? 61

What Are The Cyberknife® Robotic System and Hypofractionated Radiotherapy? 62

*Proton-beam Therapy vs. DART With Brachytherapy:
Which Is Best For Treating Prostate Cancer?* 65

The Size of the Proton Beam Requires "Scattering" to treat Prostate Cancer 67

Protons Versus Photons: Which Is State Of The Art? 68

*How effective Is The High Energy Photon Beam Used In DART /
4D IG-IMRT Compared to The Proton Beam?* 69

What the Research on Protons Tells Us 70

What Is Neutron Beam Therapy And How Does It Compare With Other Forms of Radiation? 71

What are the Treatment Options if External Radiation Fails? 73

What are the Treatment Options if Brachytherapy Fails? 74

What are the Treatment Options if Combined Radiotherapy Fails? 75

APPENDICES

A: Dr. Dattoli on the Case for Brachytherapy 77

B: State of the Art Brachytherapy, IMRT and DART 81

C: A Summary of 16-year Data 85

D: Survey Comparing Primary Treatment Modalities 89

E: Deciding What is Best for You 91

F: Glossary of Medical Terms 93

G: The Warning Signs of Prostate Cancer 107

About the Author 108

The Dattoli Cancer Foundation Mission 109

Order More Booklets in the Series 110

INTRODUCTION

THE ESSENTIAL TOOLS FOR FIGHTING PROSTATE CANCER

Having spent more than thirty years studying prostate cancer and treating more than ten thousand men, I am well aware of the controversies in this field of medicine, including when to treat and when not to treat this disease. Prostate cancer is one of the most commonly diagnosed forms of cancer, with the American Cancer Society estimating that approximately 268.490 men will be diagnosed with prostate cancer in 2021. The good news is that unlike other cancers, such as lung cancer or colon cancer, prostate cancer is typically more curable.

While we are learning more each day, there are still unsolved mysteries and many conflicting viewpoints about this disease. Some prostate cancers are rather indolent and slow-growing and may not require treatment, while others are rapidly spreading and potentially lethal, usually calling for some form of treatment. Some prostate cancer tumors make themselves known by driving up prostatic specific antigen (PSA) levels in the blood, while others lurk in the gland without raising the PSA red flag and can only be identified through skilled digital examination and/or highly sophisticated technologies such as 3D Color-Flow Power Doppler Ultrasound and Multiparametric MRI (magnetic resonance imaging). Determining which prostate cancers are aggressive and life-threatening is crucial in deciding which patients should be treated.

What is a man to do in the face of the ongoing debates as to the value of PSA screening? My advice is to heed the recommendations of the American Cancer Society, the National Cancer Institute, and other mainstream organizations addressing prostate cancer issues: Consult your personal physician and consider having an annual prostate exam by a board-certified internist or urologist, beginning at age 50 (age 45 or earlier if there is a family history of prostate cancer or if the man is African-American). The exam should include both the PSA blood test and a digital rectal exam.

If your doctor suspects you may have prostate cancer, the only way to be sure is by undergoing a prostate biopsy and having a pathologist examine tissue samples. Make sure your doctor takes at least 12 core samples in the biopsy—the more samples, the better your chance will be of obtaining an accurate result. With regard to diagnosis and treatment, it is often wise to obtain second opinions from one or more specialists within the field, keeping in mind that each specialist is likely to be biased to some degree toward his or her own particular treatment specialty.

If you are diagnosed with prostate cancer, give yourself time to evaluate ALL your treatment options. Don't make a panicked, knee-jerk decision while still in the shock of hearing your diagnosis. We are fortunate to live at a time when there are a number of effective treatment options for this disease. These include Dynamic Adaptive Radiotherapy (DART), which utilizes all the modalities associated with 4-Dimensional Image-Guided Intensity Modulation Therapy (4D IG-IMRT), and brachytherapy (pronounced brak-e-therapy). This highly effective treatment protocol is the subject of this booklet.

These sophisticated types of radiation therapy are relatively noninvasive and have profoundly improved our ability to maintain quality of life for patients. In addition, thanks to these therapeutic innovations, we are now able to successfully treat even high risk patients (those with high PSA values, high Gleason scores, and locally advanced cancer).

As you investigate your treatment options, depending on the specifics of your case, weigh the pros and cons of each type of therapy for which you are a candidate. And ask your doctor the hard questions about any treatment you may consider: *"How many men have you treated with this therapy? How many have a profile similar to mine? What are the published success rates of this therapy? What are your success rates?"* It is also wise to seek out other men who have been treated for prostate cancer. You may benefit by attending one of the Us TOO International prostate cancer information and support meetings, or other such groups in your area. By gathering all of the relevant facts that you can, you will be able to make a more fully informed treatment decision.

I strongly encourage you to work with your doctor and become an integral, proactive part of that decision-making process. As you conduct your research, be cautious about what you read in the news media and consider the sources. There are many misconceptions about prostate cancer that find their way into the media, including many of the popular medical websites and blogs on the Internet. Remember that just because something is "new" doesn't mean that it is better or has been proven to be effective. You will want to place your confidence—and your life and quality of life after treatment—in the hands of an experienced physician who can show you his or her long-term track record treating prostate cancer.

INTRODUCTION: PRECISION RADIATION THERAPY AND PROSTATE CANCER

In my practice, which for many years has been in large part devoted to radiation therapy and prostate cancer, I want my patients to be very comfortable with their treatment. The patient who has become informed and knows what to anticipate will come through his treatment with more practical knowledge and greater peace of mind.

In the past, radical surgery was considered "The Gold Standard" treatment for prostate cancer; but in recent years the evidence-based data shows virtually no advantage and many disadvantages with surgery compared to other forms of treatment. Sometimes I can tell that a man is not going to be comfortable with any treatment other than one of the surgical options. Some men have that mindset. When I sense that is the case, I may tell him that if his test results predict that his cancer is still confined to the prostate gland, perhaps he can undergo surgery if he is so inclined. In discussing treatment options with patients, I try to be as even-keeled as possible, knowing that the choice is ultimately theirs to make. At the same time, I want each patient to be aware as much as possible of the peer-reviewed results published in the field by the leading practitioners of each type of treatment.

I find that the evidence-based data often speaks for itself. While it may sound very logical to say, "You have a cancer, and we should cut it out," this option may not be so attractive if the patient is also informed that even in the best surgical hands, there is a high probability that some cancer will be left behind after surgery, that there is a risk he may have to wear diapers for the rest of his life, and there is a strong likelihood that he will suffer from erectile dysfunction. Armed with this additional information based on the most recent surgical data, the patient may want to think very hard about his choice and at least consider other options. In the end, whatever he decides, each man should feel confident that he has made the right choice for himself based on his own particular needs and individual case.

The purpose of this booklet is to provide patients considering the combined treatment regimen of DART and brachytherapy with the most up to date and accurate information to help guide you from diagnosis to recovery. Before making any decisions about treatment, you should carefully evaluate the likelihood of cure for each treatment option and the risk of side effects that may alter your quality of life. Taking into account your age, overall health, and the extent and aggressiveness of the cancer, you will want to find a balance between treatment effectiveness and potential side effects—a balance with which you are comfortable and can live with before, during and after treatment. Regardless of the type of therapy you decide is right for you, having a positive mental outlook and knowing what to expect each step of the way are keys to winning the fight against this disease.

–Michael J. Dattoli, M.D.

OVERVIEW

IMRT WITH DART AND BRACHYTHERAPY

What is Radiation and How Does It Work?

X-ray radiation is a form of energy similar to visible light. When directed at the body, x-rays penetrate tissue and are gradually absorbed. Some of the radiation is absorbed by cells and damages the DNA that normally allows cells to function and reproduce. Cancer cells are somewhat more sensitive to radiation than are healthy cells, and therefore, the radiation used to destroy cancer cells is less likely to damage normal tissues, which are tenacious. However, this difference in sensitivity is generally small and the dose of radiation required to destroy prostate cancer cells is high enough that there is some risk of damage to healthy tissue in the nearby rectum or bladder.

The strategy with radiation therapy over the years has been to deliver higher and higher doses more and more accurately to the targeted cancer, while sparing healthy adjacent tissue in order to avoid rectal and urinary complications. Radiation is measured by a unit called the Gray (Gy), roughly analogous to a Watt of light. Radiotherapists often describe radiation dose rates in terms of centigray (cGy), or 100 Gray units (what used to be called a "rad").

Since the 1950s, radiation therapy (RT) in various forms has been a common technique used for the treatment of many kinds of cancers. It is a standard treatment for prostate cancer that is clinically confined to the prostate and surrounding tissues (stages T1, T2, and T3). It may also be prescribed for patients with prostate cancer that has spread to the pelvic lymph nodes. Patients with advanced prostate cancer may also be treated with external radiation as a palliative (non-curative) therapy to reduce the size of the tumor and alleviate symptoms.

Radiation therapy has a long history dating back a century, but recent developments in treating cancer with radiation have achieved goals that were unimaginable to pioneers in the field. Progress in the field is based on modern developments in physics, mathematics and computer science, engineering, radiation delivery, diagnostic imaging, and molecular biology. Technological innovations have made possible increasingly precise delineation of tumors and their microscopic extensions, and 4-dimensional radiation delivery that takes into account organ motion with avoidance of normal tissues.

It should be noted that radiation can be delivered either continuously, as is the case with brachytherapy (radioactive seed implantation), or with fractionated sessions, as is the case with external beam radiation therapy. The dose of radiation delivered varies with the different radiotherapy modalities utilized. With fractionated radiation delivery, patients typically undergo a number of treatment sessions in order to receive the prescribed dose.

Patients with a limited number of metastases (lymph nodes and/or bone) have what is known as Oligometastic disease, and these patients may benefit from DART in order to take these areas of disease out of the equation. Our ability to visualize these areas so we can aim at them has greatly improved in recent years. We believe we are giving these patients an additional lease on life and allowing them to preserve their quality of life as long as possible.

What is External Beam Radiation Therapy?

With the conventional approach known as external beam radiation therapy (EBRT), high energy X-rays are targeted directly to the region of the prostate in order to kill or incapacitate any cancer cells in the area. The machine most widely used today to administer EBRT is the linear accelerator, which uses electrical principles (electrons) to generate photon radiation. The linear accelerator has replaced an older generation of machines that utilized radioactive cobalt and were not nearly as accurate.

Radiation is given to the patient in small daily doses, usually five days a week over a course of 6 to 8 weeks (30 to 40 treatment sessions). Delivering small, incremental doses over time decreases the chance of damaging healthy tissue. Radiation is completely painless and cannot be felt by the patient. A single treatment can be carried out in several minutes. A typical daily dose of external radiation may range from about 180 to 200 cGy.

In the past, with conventional EBRT, a patient would undergo a treatment planning session, during which the patient's lower abdomen and pelvic area was scanned with either CT scans or MRI scans to carefully determine the size and position of the patient's prostate. The radiotherapy team would then construct a system to hold the patient in the same physical position in relation to the radiation beams for each treatment. As much as possible, the intensity and direction of the beams of radiation were set to conform to the size, shape, position of the patient's prostate based on the initial CT or MRI scans.

With today's more advanced technology, preparation for external beam radiation therapy is a more rigorously complex process that involves exact determination of the region to receive treatment and the appropriate dose of radiation. Radiation treatments are precisely designed for each patient, because each man's prostate and surrounding organs are unique in size and shape. A planning session is carried out with the patient several days before treatments begin. In order to keep the patient in the same position for each daily treatment, the AlignRT system allows the radiation technologist to know exactly where the patient is at all time, before and during treatment. AlignRT utilizes a highly sophisticated 3D stereo camera system that creates an external map of the body in the set-up position and then monitors the skin surface in real time with submillimeter accuracy before and during treatment. Once the patient's body is properly aligned, fluoroscopic, computerized tomography ("Cone Beam Helical Tomography"), and ultrasound imaging techniques are used to visualize the prostate and nearby organs. With the most sophisticated radiotherapy, even respiratory acquisition video ("Respiratory Gating") is utilized to account for small movement associated with breathing ("pelvic breathing"). The position of these critical structures will determine where the radiation beams should be directed and also the shape of the beams.

The tools described above allow thorough evaluation of the 4th dimension (motion) prior to and during treatment. Adjustments are constantly made as required. These leading edge techniques are known as Adaptive Radiation Therapy (ART) or Dynamic Adaptive Radiation Therapy (DART). During treatment, beams from several directions converge to form a high-dose target zone, which includes the prostate and a margin of tissue surrounding the gland. The radiation can be focused on the target area while minimizing the risk of over-radiating the rectum and bladder.

What are the Risks of Side Effects with External Radiation?

As with radical prostatectomy, there are possible side effects with conventional external beam radiation therapy. Common side effects are fatigue, urinary urgency, frequency and burning on urination, and rectal irritation. The majority of these symptoms will disappear after treatment is concluded, but in some cases damage to the bladder or, less frequently, to the rectum results in chronic complications. These include urethral and bladder inflammation and the need to urinate more frequently (urethritis, cystitis), and intermittent periods of rectal bleeding or rectal urgency that may continue for years afterwards. Severe bladder or rectal injury is very rare. Although most men retain erectile function after the conclusion of the most advanced forms of radiation therapy, as many as half of the men who undergo older, conventional EBRT will eventually develop erectile dysfunction.

The skill of the radiotherapist administering treatments can significantly reduce the risk of complications, as can the use of more advanced technology. Conventional EBRT has largely been replaced in this country by more sophisticated techniques for delivering radiation. As discussed below, 3-D Conformal Radiation Therapy and Intensity Modulated Radiation Therapy have shown superior results both for curing the cancer and reducing the likelihood of complications. Dynamic Adaptive Radiotherapy (DART) utilizing all the technology associated with 4 Dimensional Image Guided Intensity Modulated Radiation Therapy (4D IG-IMRT) is the most advanced form of IMRT currently available.

What is 3D-Conformal Radiation Therapy?

In the past, some researchers suggested that radiation therapy might only halt progression of the disease for a number of years, after which the cancer would recur. But many radiotherapists argued that this was only the case if the radiation beam was imprecisely directed during treatment and thus failed to deliver a sufficient cancer-killing dose. Until the mid-1980's, the maximum dose that could be safely administered to the prostate was thought to be 7000 cGy. Higher doses at that time were associated with an unacceptably high risk of complications. With the improved technologies in use today, doses of 7000 to 8500 cGy are common with the technique known as 3D-Conformal Radiation (3D-CRT), which has greatly reduced the risk of complications.

Since the mid-1980's, three-dimensional computerized imaging techniques have vastly improved the accuracy of external radiation and allowed for the safe delivery of increased doses. Guided by these technological innovations, the radiotherapist molds blocks of lead alloy to conform precisely to the outline of the tumor. In order to shield healthy tissues and organs that are to be avoided, the blocks are clamped to the end of the linear accelerator, and by this means, the radiation treatment is precisely tailored for each individual patient.

Long term results of ten years and longer with 3D-Conformal Radiation Therapy have been very favorable. Because of the increased accuracy, side effects of conformal radiation are less common than with the traditional application of external beam radiation therapy. In addition, the increased dose delivered by 3D-CRT increased cure rates to a point comparable to those achieved with surgery. Yet even this relatively advanced technique for delivering external radiation has been surpassed and replaced by cutting edge modalities such as Intensity Modulated Radiation Therapy and brachytherapy.

What is Intensity Modulated Radiation Therapy?

Intensity Modulated Radiation Therapy (IMRT) is currently the state of the art when it comes to external radiation therapy, taking 3D-CRT to an even higher level of precision and control. With IMRT, the single beam of radiation is replaced by thousands of "beamlets" or "micro-beams," each with its own intensity and energy level as directed by the radiotherapist. A unique treatment blueprint is mapped out in advance for each patient.

With computer planning and three-dimensional imaging techniques, the physician is able to more accurately deliver radiation to satisfy pre-defined dose specifications to the tumor while avoiding nearby healthy tissue. Thus, the risk of damaging the bowel, bladder, rectum and other organs is significantly reduced. At the same time, the cancer-killing dose of radiation is maximized on the designated target (see Color Images 6–9).

As noted, at our center, we offer the most sophisticated form of IMRT, known as **4-Dimensional Image-Guided Intensity Modulated Radiation Therapy (4D IG-IMRT) with Dynamic Adaptive Radiotherapy (DART)**. This multifaceted modality utilizes a number of advanced targeting and imaging techniques even beyond what was available just a few years ago with the first generation of IMRT. The 4th dimension refers to motion and our ability to track motion (patient and organ movement) thanks in part to enhanced imaging and computer programming capabilities.

4D-IG IMRT represents the latest generation of IMRT, with the most exquisite control of treatment microbeams. When combining multiple 4D technologies (at least 5) modalities, an unprecedented level of precision is realized with DART.

The references to IMRT in the sections immediately ahead generally apply to the entire range of technologies currently being used, including 4D IG-IMRT (or 4D IGRT), which utilizes a number of technical refinements, which will be discussed in greater detail below (see "What is Dynamic Adaptive Radiotherapy (DART)?" and "What are the 4D IG-IMRT Analysis Tools for Image Guidance to Achieve DART?").

How is IMRT Planned and Performed?

With IMRT, each treatment volume is considered on a voxel by voxel basis (with a voxel being a cubic millimeter of space) and each voxel may receive a different dose. This is like treating an area the size of a tip of a pen. Once the "target" has been designated, a planning phase referred to as "inverse treatment planning" generates beam profiles with varying intensities across the treatment field. The intensity profile of each beamlet is adjusted to satisfy the predefined dose specifications to the tumor as well as to the normal tissues. A computer, using mathematical optimization algorithms, then runs the optimization program, which selects the best combination of directions and beam intensities to obtain the ideal optimized plan. The program consists of literally thousands of discreet angles and doses.

To accomplish the planning phase, extremely sophisticated computerized software is utilized and plans are generated in a time frame measured in hours. This task might take a world class physicist years to accomplish. Since we are generating high-energy beamlets at specific cubic millimeter targets, immobilization of the patient is imperative. For this reason, a number of checks and balances are put into place prior to and during treatment.

Once the patient's treatment profile has been digitally reconstructed, and a specific program or blueprint for that patient is developed, verification of the IMRT treatment is performed by utilizing amorphous silicone diode imaging, which is referred to as "Portal Vision." This silicon diode has unprecedented resolution and image acquisition, so that the doctor can watch the treatment in "real time," or review this program at the workstation at a later time. The actual delivery of the radiation is a dynamic process and is accomplished through the use of multi-leaf collimators. These devices essentially allow us to "sculpt" the beams in order to deliver the precise dose required.

What is Dynamic Adaptive Radiotherapy (DART)?

For more than four decades, the evolution of radiation delivery technologies has been based upon a single objective: maximize the dose to the tumor while minimizing the dose to surrounding normal tissue (thereby minimizing side effects). As noted previously, today the most advanced beam technology available is known as high resolution 4-Dimensional Image-Guided Intensity Modulated Radiation Therapy (4D IG-IMRT), also referred to as 4D-IGRT. The Dattoli Cancer Center was the first private facility in America to offer it to patients. Using 4D IG-IMRT, we are able to realize the full potential of what is known as Dynamic Adaptive Radiotherapy (DART).

4D-IG IMRT represents the latest generation of IMRT, with the most exquisite control of treatment micro-beams. When combining multiple 4D technologies (at least 5), an unprecedented level of precision is realized with DART.

As implemented at our center, DART is a coordinated systems approach made possible by the technological convergence of image-guided tools, which integrate both image and data management while utilizing sophisticated treatment planning capabilities such as "autosegmentation" and "deformable registration" – all for the purpose of optimized 4D IG-IMRT treatment delivery. Such a cutting edge system ties together every step, from 4D IG-IMRT simulation and treatment planning to adaptive treatment delivery based on the reality of a patient's exact treatment condition and position each and every day even as it changes. It is becoming increasingly well known that changes such as tumor position, size and shape occur not only during a several week treatment regime, but also on a daily basis.

DART has been refined at the Dattoli Cancer Center as the most sophisticated form of external radiation beam therapy currently available. It is superior to all previous generations of Intensity Modulated Radiotherapy (IMRT), Image-Guided Radiation Therapy (IGRT) and 3D Conformal Radiation Therapy (3DCRT). DART incorporates every device used for 4D Image-Guided IMRT, taking it to a new level of precision and control. This increased level of accuracy allows us to shoot microbeams or beamlets of radiation to targets the size of grains of sand. As noted, these volumes are referred to as "voxels." Each voxel is a cubic millimeter. This degree of pinpoint control and focus enables us to target the cancer while greatly reducing the risk of damage to the bowel and bladder, as well as preserving erectile function in most cases.

A unique treatment blueprint is mapped out in advance for each patient. The actual implementation of DART relies on handling large volumes of continuously changing patient data, interpreting those changes and then immediately acting upon them in real-time. For example, rather than using a one-size-fits-all approach, physicians are empowered to choose a dose schema (e.g. "boost") at a chosen moment in time and make necessary changes to a treatment plan "on the fly" based on Cone Beam image capture that reveals real-time changes in the target as it responds to treatment. The bottom line involves managing the motion and biological changes of the target (tumor) and dynamically adapting the 4D IG-IMRT treatment. This makes for truly individualized treatment delivery.

Even the simple motion of breathing can shift the position of the prostate. But we can track, anticipate and correct for physiologic movement by our special 2nd generation Respiratory Gating System. This is an advanced video tracking technology that allows for real-time monitoring that accounts for patient breathing. Included in the DART suite are strict immobilization techniques utilizing Vac-Lock assistance, motion sensing tracking cameras, and AlignRT surface guidance, along with Varian Exact Couch™ and PortalVision™ with Exact Arm positioning.

A unique ensemble of cutting edge technologies—electronic online portal imaging ("portal vision" and "portal dosimetry"), electronic on-board portal imaging, 4th generation Cone Beam Tomography and real-time 4D soft tissue and bone to bone matching capability add another crucial layer of accuracy checks that ensure a level of precision not dreamed of just five years ago.

In order to make sure that each microbeam reaches the designated target, the 4th dimension of motion must be taken into account. All the components of DART enable us to deliver the right dose to the right target at precisely the right time—each time and every time. Based on physiological and anatomical changes that occur between individual treatments and during each treatment, our physicians, physicists, dosimetrists, therapists and combination of technical equipment can modulate or alter the original treatment plan to account for these daily changes. This highly integrated approach is the key to DART—intra- and inter-fractional adjustments allowing for the most precise targeting of tumor(s) imaginable.

It should be noted that with DART not only is the prostate tracked, but also specific areas within the prostate are tracked as are all of the critical surrounding tissues (e.g. bladder, rectum, neurovascular bundles, uro-genital diaphragm, ano-rectal penile bulb, penile crus). Moreover, during the tracking, microbeams are dynamically adjusted to reach their designated target (like "smart missiles"). Typically, patients will receive 8000 to 9000 cGy to the target area, and the urethra will get approximately 20% less. The tumors, depending on where they are located, will be anywhere from 8% to 20% hotter. There are cases where the dose is 30% or even 40% higher, but those are unusual. And we can do that without any undue side effects.

When DART is utilized as a monotherapy, patients receive daily 4D IG-IMRT treatments over 6 to 8 weeks, Monday through Friday (30 to 40 sessions). Each treatment is approved by the doctors with the aid of amorphous silicon diodes (portal vision), and reviewed by the physician in real time using a unique wireless network.

With our combined protocol, after completion of the DART sessions, many patients return in 10 days to 8 weeks for brachytherapy (seed implantation) as described later in this booklet, if their risk factors mandate a combined approach. Approximately 90 days after the seed implant procedure, patients may also receive a short, follow-up course of 8 to 10 additional "boost" DART treatments to sterilize any microscopic cancer that might have invaded the periprostatic tissues or lymph nodes of the pelvis and/or abdomen.

What are the 4D IG-IMRT Analysis Tools for Image Guidance to Achieve DART?

As noted above, daily localization of the target is essential to optimize therapeutic effects since both patient and organ movement may occur. It should be noted that all of the following 4D IG-IMRT Analysis Tools are non-invasive. These routines are implemented with comprehensive checklists that are crucial to ensure accurate targeting on a daily basis. The integration of these state-of-the-art technologies makes DART possible and allows our physicians to maximize the radiation dose to the tumor while minimizing the dose to surrounding normal tissue, thereby minimizing side effects.

Strict Immobilization Techniques using Vac-Lock, tracking cameras and the table, which is called the "exact couch." There are tracking cameras located within the treatment head which is called the "exact arm." If there is more than a millimeter of motion, that will be sensed and a default will come into play.

SpaceOAR Technique creates a temporary space between the rectum and the prostate gland, enabling us to target radiation to the prostate while sparing healthy tissue. OAR stands for "organ at risk," refer-ring to the rectum. With ultrasound guidance, a hydrogel is injected through the perineum. It solidifies, creating an approximate 1 cm space between the prostate and the rectum.

Electronic Online Portal Imaging ("Portal Vision") using amorphous silicon diode technology which allows for real-time on-line verification of patient's exact treatment plan. This is an eloquent way of looking at the patient in real time.

Portal Dosimetry allows us to identify if the patient has changed or if there is motion during the treatment period. We invest considerable time, energy and technology to create a "virtual you," a true image of you that is an accurate blueprint. If Portal Imaging shows a change, then Portal Dosimetry will automatically re-optimize your treatment plan.

Electronic On-Board Imaging for real-time evaluation. This involves what is known as 3rd and 4th dimensional bone-to-bone and soft tissue matching.

4th Generation Cone Beam Tomography involves real-time helical CT anatomical reconstruction of patient's anatomy to determine the actual daily delivered dose for adaptive radiotherapy. This is an actual CT Cone Beam activated while the patient is being treated. We have a wireless real time system that enables physicians to watch what is happening with the patient in real time. If anything appears inappropriate we are able to manually override the program. So there is still a decisive human touch to all of this advanced technology.

It should be noted that Cone Beam CT ("Tomo Therapy") is not the same as "tomotherapy." The latter is actually a form of radiation treatment delivered using CT guidance, both of which are continuous in nature and very slow (rotational arc). The patient is often treated for 40 minutes so that the "BEAM-ON TIME" is enormous. This leads to "incident planned radiation," which then has a high integral dose because of the arc and the duration of treatment, with scattered photons and neutrons from the planned incident radiation, and the radiation from a continuously revolving CT Scan, which can also impart a sizeable dose to the entire body. As such, with this form of radiation treatment, there is a high risk of developing secondary cancers. Indeed, tomotherapy delivers such enormous doses of Total Body Radiation (TBR) that it is not recommended in pediatric cancers (patients in their twenties or less).

Why would a 50 year old or even a 60 year old patient want to undergo tomotherapy for prostate cancer only to get leukemia after 5 to 10 years? In contrast, at our institution, we use "light speed" CT scans for diagnostics, which is accomplished in seconds. Our Cone Beam CT is also a "light speed" helical scanner so that the radiation dose is quantifiable although small and safe. The problem is that Cone Beam CT is often referred to as "Cone Beam CT Tomo Therapy," but it is really Cone Beam (CB) Tomography. It is not a form of treatment, but just one of our many image guidance tools used in conjunction with 4D IG-IMRT and DART.

Real-time 4D review by physicians using wireless network system which conveys images to remote tablet.

2nd Generation Respiratory Gating is another way that we can identify patient motion, with advanced video tracking technology which allows for real-time monitoring and correction of physiologic motion of the prostate which may occur as a result of patient breathing. It should be noted that DART is not possible without Respiratory Gating; and most centers do not offer this technology as it is prohibitively expensive.

AlignRT is a tracking system that facilitates what is known as Surface Guided Radiation Therapy (SGRT), tracking patient motion and complementing the Respiratory Gating program. AlignRT assists in the initial placement of the patient on the exact couch, and to monitor and manage movement during the treatment period to a pre-set tolerance level.

While patients are very compliant in trying to remain still during the treatment period, sometimes an involuntary movement occurs – a sneeze, for instance. With

AlignRT, real time tracking of patient movement is detected and the treatment machine will automatically hold the beam, reset the patient position and then restart the treatment without having the therapist re-enter the room.

The AlignRT system delivers high precision positioning and movement monitoring that contributes to patient safety from over- or under-dosing of radiation, reduces time when movement is detected, and reduces unnecessary possible exposure to radiation for the therapist. AlignRT also eliminates the necessity for placement tattoos!

CT SIM+™ with RapidSIM™ is the most recent addition to our arsenal of DART analysis tools for image guidance.

This modality allows for deformable fusion between our CT workstations and other diagnostic technologies such as 3D Color-Flow Power Doppler Ultrasound and Multiparametric MRI. This modality makes for highly accurate treatment planning, delineating specific targets for macroscopic tumor dose escalation and dose reduction to microscopic targets.

This high-precision approach to curing cancer has been the dream of radiation therapy dating back more than four decades. The equipment is continually updated from first generation models to more refined succeeding generation enhanced by further innovations.

How Does IMRT Compare to 3D-CRT?

A number of recent studies comparing IMRT to 3D-CRT have demonstrated a very significant advantage for IMRT with respect to both success rates and reduction of side effects. One study from Memorial Sloan-Kettering showed IMRT increased the success rate in shrinking tumors from 43% to 96%, while decreasing complications from 10% to 2%. Our team and others are reporting similar findings.

As we will see in the pages ahead, 4D IG IMRT (or 4D-IGRT) offers even greater advantages when it is combined with brachytherapy, especially with intermediate and high risk patients. It should also be noted that 4D IG-IMRT is not considered an experimental procedure, but is rather the culmination of earlier external radiation delivery systems. Like brachytherapy, all of the modalities and imaging techniques associated with 4D IG-IMRT are FDA and Medicare approved, and its effectiveness has already been demonstrated by many scientific studies.

Keep in mind that with the rapid advances in IMRT and related technologies, not all IMRT is created equal. Many institutions advertize that they offer "IMRT" when in fact they have only early generations of this technology that is not adaptive. *Patients are strongly advised to make sure their doctors are equipped with the latest IMRT technology, or 4D IG-IMRT with DART.* By taking the time to locate which medical centers in their area have state of the art technology, patients are more likely to have successful outcomes. Many patients travel to our center from around the world simply because we have the most advanced technology and we are continually upgrading to maintain the highest standards.

As noted, conventional IMRT is fractionated, typically given to the patient in small daily doses (fractions), usually five days a week over 8 to 10 weeks. Delivering small, incremental doses over time decreases the chance of damaging healthy tissue. With moderately hypofractionated IMRT, larger doses are administered over a much shorter period of time, often 4 to 6 weeks. With extreme, ultra-hypofractionated radiotherapy, the dose is even higher and the duration of treatment is even shorter (5-6 fractions or fewer).

The majority of studies suggest that acute and late side effects are likely to be higher with hypofractionated IMRT than with conventional IMRT. Acute toxicity results in long-term injury to surrounding, healthy tissues (i.e. rectum, bladder, urethra. Neurovascular bundles and other critical neighboring structures).

The published guidelines of the American Society of Clinical Oncology recommend that physicians should counsel patients about the limited follow-up beyond five years for most studies evaluating hypofractionation and the increased risk of acute and late toxicity with Moderately Hypofractionated IMRT compared to Conventional IMRT. The guidelines suggest Ultra-Hypofractionated Radiotherapy should be limited to clinical trials due to the risk of late toxicity (Morgan SC, Hypofractionated Radiation Therapy for Localized Prostate Cancer: Executive Summary of an ASTRO, ASCO, and AUA Evidence-Based Guideline, Pract Radiat Oncol, 2018 Nov–Dec;8(6):354-360).

Which Patients are Eligible for External Radiation Therapy?

Because external radiation (including EBRT, 3D-CRT, IMRT, and DART) is non-invasive and does not require an operation or anesthesia, most men can safely tolerate this form of therapy. The likelihood of cure is greatest with low risk patients (clinical stage T1, non-palpable tumors, less than 50% core involvement found in the biopsy specimens, a Gleason score ≤ 6, serum PSA < 10, and a non-elevated PAP). Intermediate and high risk patients can also be effectively treated with external radiation, but more favorable results for these patients are now being achieved when external radiation is combined with brachytherapy.

With the combined protocol of DART and brachytherapy, even patients having locally advanced disease with lymph node involvement have enjoyed long disease-free intervals and even a cure. These patients were previously thought to be incurable.

In addition, patients with metastatic disease beyond the regional lymph nodes have not been considered curable in the past; however, with the most recent advances in technology, we are beginning to push the envelope with our ability to treat more advanced cases. We now treat the primary tumor, and with certain limitations, we treat all known sites of metastatic deposits to prolong the disease-free interval.

In patients having metastatic disease, when the cancer in the prostate region is causing urinary or rectal problems, they are often treated with external radiation. Patients with bone metastases may also be treated with radiation to relieve bone pain.

As noted earlier, DART utilizing all the technology associated with 4D IG-IMRT is often appropriate for those patients who may not be eligible for brachytherapy. These patients include the following:

1. A man with too large a Transurethral Resection of the Prostate (TURP) defect, or has had multiple TURPS, making the implantation of seeds inadvisable.
2. A prostate that is too large and cannot be downsized with hormones.
3. Patients with severe bladder outlet obstruction that cannot be improved with medication and/or procedures such as photoselective vaporization of the prostate (PVP).
4. Post-prostatectomy patients without enough tissue left to anchor seeds.
5. Patients who have had a previous seeding procedure that has maximized the dose to the prostate. This is somewhat rare since most of these men were under-treated with seeds (received too little radiation to the target area) which is why the disease recurred.
6. A recurrence after any form of primary treatment when no local disease is found, only distant spread. It should be noted that with recurrent cancers, patients with lower serum PSA values are more likely to be cured with DART (utilizing 4D IG-IMRT) as a salvage therapy.

What is Brachytherapy?

Brachytherapy, also called *interstitial implantation therapy*, involves the placement of tiny radioactive seeds or pellets directly into the prostate gland. The radioactive seeds can either be inserted temporarily, or can remain permanently in place within the prostate. They provide a high dose of radiation that is concentrated in the prostate. Permanent seeds pose no health threat to the patient since their radiation decays within 6 months to a year, and thereafter, they become inert.

Brachytherapy has a fairly long history. As early as 1917, a crude form of seed implantation using radium needles was performed at what is now Memorial Sloan-

Kettering Cancer Center. The chief of urology at that time, Dr. Benjamin Barringer, was so enthusiastic about the procedure that he concluded his report in the *Journal of the American Medical Association,* "... because of the initial success of radium treatment, I now take the stand that no patient with prostate cancer should be operated on."

In fact, the technology had not yet been developed that would make the procedure fully effective. The 1980's saw renewed interest in seed implants because the development of ultrasound imaging, CT scans and fluoroscopic techniques allowed for precise planning and monitoring of where the seeds should be placed. Since that time, brachytherapy has become a standard, mainstream treatment for prostate cancer that is widely available throughout the U.S.

As with external beam radiation therapy, a number of technical refinements in the seed implant procedure have led to greatly improved results and increasing popularity. In the old days (as recently as the 1970's), seed implants required major abdominal surgery. Seeds of radioactive isotopes were manually implanted into the prostate using needles, but the procedure was essentially carried out blind and achieved poor results because of a lack of precision in placing the seeds. Poor placement led to "cold" spots within the prostate gland that did not receive a sufficient dose of radiation to destroy the cancer.

In more recent years, a minimally invasive technique has been devised for implanting the seeds in the prostate without open surgery (known as "transperineal implantation"). Guided by ultrasound and fluoroscopy, the seeds are dispensed through tiny hollow needles which are inserted through the perineum (the area between the scrotum and anus). A template or grid is used to precisely guide the placement of the needles.

Ultrasound allows for real time imaging and dynamic visualization. As the technology has evolved with Color-Flow Power Doppler Ultrasound, a more precise, three-dimensional image of the prostate can be generated, and the seeds can be more accurately placed, where they will be most effective. The strategy is to target and destroy the cancer with minimal exposure to surrounding healthy tissue and organs. The computerized guidance system helps determine where the seeds should go, how deeply they should be inserted, and how strong their radiation should be (see Color Images 1-4). At our institution, we use both pre-planning and intraoperative dosimetry for optimal seed placement.

Brachytherapy with ultrasound and fluoroscopic guidance has a number of advantages over conventional external beam radiation therapy. The standard dose of radiation used with EBRT is approximately 7000 cGy, calculated to be the highest dose which is safe and well tolerated by the patient. By contrast, seed implants are placed internally to deliver radiation directly to the prostate while sparing surrounding organs. As a consequence, higher doses of radiation (exceeding 12,000 cGy) can be administered to the area of the prostate, while tumorous sites often receive doses in excess of 20,000 cGy. In addition, the radiation delivered by seeds is continuous over the time they are active, *working around the clock to kill the cancer.* By contrast, all other forms of radiation, including temporary High Dose Rate (HDR) brachytherapy, are fractionated (see Figure 1), which means the radiation is administered only in intermittent doses.

MODALITY	TYPICAL DOSE	DELIVERY
3D-CRT	7000–8500 cGy	Fractionated
IMRT (4D IG-IMRT) IGRT DART	7000–9100 cGy	Fractionated
Protons/Neutrons CyberKnife	7000–8500 cGy Dose investigational	Fractionated Fractionated
Rapid Arc Radiation	7000–9100 cGy (Radiation Dose Investigational)	Fractionated
Pd-103/I-125 Brachytherapy (Monotherapy)	12,500 cGy/14,400 cGy	Continuous
HDR Ir-192 (Monotherapy)	Dose investigational	Fractionated
All forms of EBRT and HDR Ir-192	4000–5000 cGy (EBRT-HDR) 1500–2500 cGy (Brachy-HDR)	Fractionated Fractionated
3D-CRT/IMRT (DART) and Pd-103/I-125	4000–5400 cGy *plus* 8000–12,000 cGy	Fractionated/ Continuous

Figure 1
A Comparison of radiotherapy modalities for treatment of localized (loco-regional) prostate cancer. Continuous versus Fractionated radiation therapy.

Dr. Dattoli on the Choice of Brachytherapy Isotopes

Palladium-103 and Iodine-125 are the most commonly used radioisotopes for permanent prostate brachytherapy. Neither type of seed needs to be removed from the body after implantation, as they are made from materials that are accepted by the body over time. They are non-ferromagnetic and will not interfere with diagnostic tests such as CT's or MRI's. The choice of Pd-103 versus I-125 is typically based on physician preference, though it is sometimes driven by patients. While the debate continues as to which isotope is superior, Palladium has long been my isotope of choice, even for low-grade prostate malignancies.

My preference dates back to my experience with both Pd-103 and I-125 at New York University Medical Center and Memorial Sloan-Kettering in the mid-1980s. My research and clinical practice in Tampa over the following decade and my experience in Sarasota during the past two decades have confirmed for me the advantages of Pd-103 for my patients.

While there have been no definitive human clinical trials to date comparing tumor-control rates with Pd-103 and I-125, one study reported a lower complication rate for Pd-103 (Peschel RE, et al, Cancer J. 2004 May-Jun;10(3):170-4.) Another study reported a faster recovery rate from radiation-induced prostatitis with Pd-103 (Wallner K, et al, Cancer J. 2002 Jan-Feb;8(1):67-73).

Both Palladium and Iodine are effective implant sources, but I have found the short-lived side effects associated with Pd-103 to be especially advantageous in the context of a large brachytherapy-based practice. The following discussion is not intended to settle the debate, but rather to explain my rationale over the years for encouraging my patient to choose Pd-103.

The radiobiology and dose rate phenomenon of Pd-103 versus I-125 have been rigorously studied. A Pd-103 implant is usually planned to deliver a 11,500-12,000 cGy to full decay at an initial dose rate of approximately 20 cGy/hour. I-125 implants deliver radiation at a lower dose rate of approximately 5-10 cGy/hour. The half-life for each isotope is the period of time until its output of radiation is halved. The half-life of Pd-103 is seventeen days compared to sixty days with I-125. With Palladium, most of the radiation dosage is delivered in three months compared to six to eight months with Iodine. While the dose delivery is as stated, side effects with each isotope may be longer in duration due to clinical lag time.

Results favoring Palladium might be expected given radiobiological considerations. Most radiobiologic data is derived from theory or based on in vitro studies. It is known that radiobiological effect (RBE) decreases with decreasing dose rate primarily as a result of the tumor's ability to repair potentially lethal and sub-lethal damage, but also because of recruitment of a relatively quiescent sub-population of cells and re-population of initial target cell populations; If the dose rate is too low, tumors associated with rapid cell cycles (e.g. 2-5 days) may not be effectively killed. Although no human clinical data with long-term follow-up is available, the higher dose rate of Pd-103 would theoretically be more successful in eradicating aggressive and rapidly proliferating tumors.

In this regard, it should be noted that low energy photons have a higher linear energy transfer (LET), associated with higher RBE. The greater radiobiologic effect is presumably the outcome of greater energy delivered per cell that the photon traverses. The average energy of Pd-103 photons is 21 keV (kiloelectron volts) as compared to 29 keV with I-125. Thus Palladium would be expected to have a slightly higher LET and RBE compared to Iodine.

In vivo animal models (e.g. studies of rat prostate tumors) and also in vitro studies do in fact demonstrate a significant benefit with Pd-103 for higher-grade tumors, but also an advantage in low-grade tumors. An early study by Nag and colleagues demonstrated the tumoricidal effect of Pd-103 was greater than I-125 by at least factor of two (Nag S, et al, J Brachyther Int. 1997; 13: 243-251). The RBE of Pd-103 versus I-125 was compared by Ling and colleagues using rat embryo cells transfected with Ha-ras oncogene. While the applicability of results from such in vitro experiments to the clinic is limited, this study reported an RBE of 1.9 for Palladium versus 1.4 for Iodine (Ling CC, The relative biological effectiveness of I-125 and Pd-103. Int J Radiat Oncol Biol Phys, 1995; 32: 373-378). These favorable Pd-103 results may be based at least in part on the dose rate phenomenon.

Only one early study suggested that I-125 might be more effective for low-grade tumors while Pd-103 would be superior for high-grade carcinomas (Ling CC, Permanent implants using Au-198, Pd-103 and I-125: Radiobiological considerations based on the linear quadratic model, Int J Radiat Oncol Biol Phys. 1992; 23: 81-87). This was a highly theoretical model based on the biologic effective dose (BED) formula, with questionable alpha/beta ratio assumptions. The study has virtually no clinical applicability, as the central mathematical

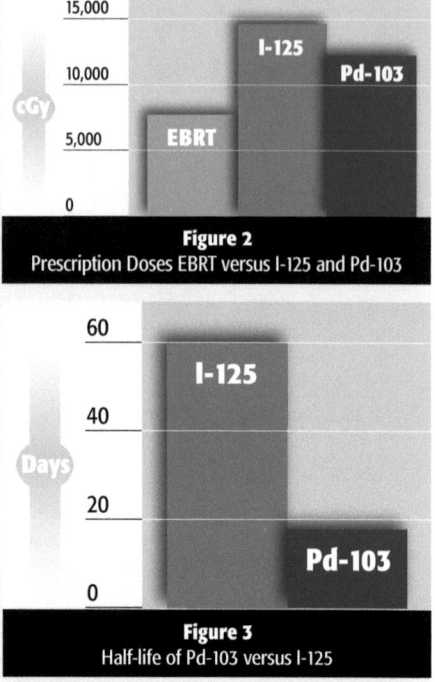

Figure 2
Prescription Doses EBRT versus I-125 and Pd-103

Figure 3
Half-life of Pd-103 versus I-125

equation used to calculate the cell survival level relied on variables about which little or nothing is known when applied to human prostate cancer.

It should be noted that a dose of 16,000 cGy with I-125 is considered biologically equivalent to a dose of 11,500 cGy with Pd-103. However, it should be understood that most I-125 dosimetry in past years used an incorrect 'gamma factor' which overestimated the dose. Therefore, when the 11,500 cGy Palladium dose is delivered, it is actually a greater radiobiological dose than was delivered by the older I-125 implants cited in the medical literature.

Because of the lower energy of photons emitted by Pd-103 compared to I-125 (21 keV avg. versus 28 keV avg.) radial dose fall-off is more steep at any distance from Pd-103 seeds, especially since attenuation coefficients (e.g., tissue, scatter, other seeds) increase rapidly with decreasing photon energy and are in fact exponential. Therefore, at greater distance from a Pd-103 implant, the dose is significantly reduced when compared to I-125, e.g., at a distance of 10 em in tissue, the dose of Pd-103 is approximately 1/10 that for I-125 (Nath R, Int J Radiat Oncol Biol Phys, 1992; 22: 1131-1138). This is not insignificant clinically and shows that tissue penetration is distinctly dissimilar between the two isotopes despite their energies being relatively similar. The same phenomenon, however, may lend itself to cold spots if Palladium seeds are not accurately placed, so an experienced brachytherapist is required to achieve optimal outcomes.

As mentioned, I have extensive experience using both Iodine and Palladium for prostate cancer (as well as Iridium-192 with High Dose Rate (HDR) temporary brachytherapy as discussed below. Both Pd-103 and I-125 cause their share of temporary urinary symptoms, but I have found the duration to be different with each isotope, while the peak severity of each is essentially the same. The peak with I-125 is slightly greater; 2-3 weeks peak for Pd-103, and 3-5 months peak for I-125.

Over the years I encountered too many patients having long-lasting, lingering symptoms with I-125, and this was somewhat discouraging. In contrast, Pd-103 symptoms are typically short-lived, predictable and I find more easily manageable: With formalized management protocols, we have significantly reduced implant morbidity. The need for catheterization in any patient is less than 2%. The faster clinical response rate associated with Pd-103 generally enables the success of treatment to be assessed more quickly.

Because of the unique concave design of the Palladium seeds, they are very stable within the gland tissue, rarely migrating outside the desired placement. By contrast, the convex (football) shape of Iodine seeds can cause them to migrate from the target. For this reason I-125 is usually inserted as "strands" which secure one seed to the next, although this leaves behind more foreign bodies and makes intra-operative changes which are almost always necessary more difficult. Iodine is a much more penetrating radiation than is Pd-103, potentially adversely affecting the bladder, urethra, rectum and sexual function.

In the unfortunate event of a prolonged catheterization with a Pd-103 implant, a transurethral incision of the prostate (TUIP) or transurethral resection of the prostate (TURP) can be safely performed without concern of interfering with cancericidal dose delivery (if seeds are disturbed or removed) since 95% of the Palladium dose is delivered within 8 weeks. This is certainly not the case with I-125 where consideration of maintaining a catheter for a much longer period must be considered. Also, the steep dose fall-off with Pd-103 allows us to more easily perform implants in patients having previous TURP's and has also enabled us to successfully salvage patients who have previously been treated with radiation and failed.

Many of my patient's treated back in the 1990s at Memorial Sloan-Kettering Cancer Center underwent very contemporary techniques implant with I-125, yet rectal ulcerations were not uncommon (Wallner K, et al, Short-term freedom from disease progression after I-125 prostate implantation. Int J Radiat Oncol Biol Phys, 1994 Sep 30;30(2):405-9). Meanwhile not one of my patient's having Pd-103 implantation has experienced a rectal ulceration.

My data over the years suggests that Palladium is indeed very effective treating low-grade prostate tumors. It is well known that patients may be initially undergraded and many of us believe that up to 40% of patients harbor higher-grade tumors within their glands that were simply missed by initial biopsies, which is another compelling argument for the use of Pd-103.

The disadvantages with Pd-103 are primarily associated with the short half-life, which requires replacement and/or dosimetric corrections if the seeds are not used at the planning date. This rarely allows for re-utilization of the isotope. Also, technical accuracy of seed placement with Pd-103 is more demanding and requires greater skill on the part of the brachytherapist. I always recommend brachytherapy newcomers to use I-125 at first since it is far more forgiving of geographical targeting misses than Pd-103. In that regard, I believe that stricter standards need to be set by the medical community to ensure improved technical acumen; a one to two day teaching course will never suffice.

With regard to our combination protocol with external beam radiation therapy and Pd.103 brachytherapy, I often tell patients that "cancer doesn't like change," and virtually all cancers today are treated with combined modalities, including external and internal radiation such as Dynamic Adaptive Radiotherapy (DART) followed by a brachytherapy boost. This change of therapeutic approach is important with virtually every cancer, hence the common utilization of combined modality treatments in contemporary cancer medicine (e.g. chemotherapy and radiotherapy, surgery and radiotherapy, and chemo-surgery-radiation)

This discussion is not intended to end the still ongoing debate over I-125 versus Pd-103, but rather to explain for patients and colleagues my rationale for choosing Pd-103. It is my hope that with improved implant techniques, results with I-125 and Pd-103 will become generalizable. Only a well-conducted, randomized clinical trial will ultimately settle the controversy, but I think the results I have reported in my published studies are telling.

Another isotope, Cesium-131, is currently being investigated as a permanent implant. It has a shorter half-life (9.7 days) and a higher average energy (29 KeV) than both I-125 and Pd-103. This means that Cesium-131 is likely to deliver a higher dose to surrounding healthy tissue over a shorter period of time; and therefore, there is a an increased risk of complications over time. Like Gold-198 (Au-198), another isotope that was used some years ago, the shorter half-life of these isotopes with 9.7 days for Cesium-131 and 2.7 days for Au-198 makes them impractical to use in a clinical setting.

A 2018 study by the MD Anderson Cancer Center compared quality of life (QoL) outcomes following brachytherapy with Palladium, Iodine and Cesium isotopes. These researchers reported that "Cs-131 showed a statistically significant decrease in QoL regarding bowel and sexual function at 12 months compared with Pd-103" (Blanchard P, et al, Patient-reported health-related quality of life for men treated with low-dose-rate prostate brachytherapy as monotherapy with 125-iodine, 103-palladium, or 131-cesium, Brachytherapy. 2018 Mar - Apr; 17(2):265-276).

Dr. Dattoli on Treating Metastatic Disease with DART

When prostate cancer spreads beyond its original site and is no longer locally confined to the prostate gland—a process called metastasis—it marks a significant turning point in the disease for patients. For many, this diagnosis can feel overwhelming, as metastatic cancer has historically been considered incurable.

However, the landscape of advanced prostate cancer treatment has evolved significantly over the past two decades thanks to technological progress and our growing knowledge of the disease. Today, there are innovative strategies that offer patients hope for improved survival while maintaining their quality of life.

Our current understanding of metastatic prostate cancer and modern approaches to treatment that have redefined what is possible for those facing this potentially life-threatening diagnosis.

Understanding Metastatic Prostate Cancer

Metastatic prostate cancer occurs when cancer cells spread from the prostate to other parts of the body, most commonly the lymph nodes, bones, lungs, and liver. Historically, metastatic prostate cancer was treated with systemic therapies alone—such as androgen deprivation therapy (ADT) and chemotherapy—aimed at controlling cancer throughout the body. However, these approaches often left persistent cancer cells in the prostate gland itself or in localized metastatic sites, which had since become resistant to systemic agents.

As a result, these remaining cancer cells often progress and spread, leading to problems within the prostate region itself. These cancer cells are also left to colonize distant sites such as the lymph nodes, bone, lungs and liver.

A Shift in Perspective

For decades, the prevailing belief was that treating the primary tumor in cases of metastasis was futile. However, emerging evidence has challenged this view. Research now suggests that treating the prostate gland—even in the context of metastasis—can influence outcomes by reducing tumor burden and potentially slowing or preventing further spread.

One of the most intriguing concepts in this field is that of the abscopal effect. This phenomenon describes how local treatments like radiation therapy not only target tumors at their primary site of origin but also stimulate systemic immune responses that shrink untreated tumors elsewhere in the body. This discovery opened new doors for integrating local and systemic therapies for effectively managing metastatic prostate cancer.

The Evidence: Key Clinical Trials

Several landmark studies have reshaped our understanding of metastatic prostate cancer treatment:

1. The STAMPEDE Trial (2016)
This large, randomized trial demonstrated that adding radiation therapy to systemic treatments (such as ADT) provided a significant survival benefit for men with metastatic prostate cancer, and especially for those having low-volume metastatic disease. The study showed that targeting the primary tumor with radiation could improve outcomes even when metastases were present (James, ND et al, Addition of docetaxel, zoledronic acid, or both to first-line long-term hormone therapy in **prostate** cancer (**STAMPEDE**): survival results from an adaptive, multiarm, multistage, platform randomized controlled trial; Lancet, 2016 Mar 19;387(10024):1163-77).

2. The HORRAD Trial
This clinical trial explored the benefits of combining radiation therapy with ADT specifically for men with bone metastases. The results demonstrated beneficial outcomes in patients having low-volume skeletal metastases, although even treating high-volume disease with this combined approach was associated with several superior clinical and radiographic endpoints (Boevé LMS, et al, Prostate Cancer-related Events in Patients with Synchronous Metastatic Hormone-sensitive Prostate Cancer Treated with Androgen Deprivation Therapy with and Without Concurrent Radiation Therapy to the Prostate; Data from the HORRAD Trial. Eur Urol. 2024 Sep 19:S0302-2838(24)02593-4).

3. Oligometastatic Disease Concept
A concept introduced in 1995 by University of Chicago researchers Weichselbaum and Hellman, who coined the term "oligometastases," referring to cases where cancer has spread to a limited number of distant sites (typically up to five) outside the prostate. Studies suggest that patients with oligometastatic disease may achieve long-term complete remissions—or even cure—through aggressive local treatments targeting *both* the primary tumor and metastatic sites (Oligometastases. Hellman S, Weichselbaum RR. J Clin Oncol. 1995 Jan;13(1):8-10.

Modern Treatment Strategies: A Multi-Pronged Approach
The treatment of advanced prostate cancer now often involves a combination of therapies tailored to each patient's disease characteristics. Below are key components of this multi-pronged approach:

1. Treating the Primary Tumor
Radiation therapy directed at the prostate gland remains a cornerstone of definitive treatment for localized prostate cancer. By reducing the tumor burden at its

source, this approach can delay progression and minimize complications such as urinary obstruction or pelvic pain. Recent clinical trials have validated the use of local radiation to the prostate even in the metastatic setting as well.

2. Metastasis-Directed Therapy

Advances in imaging technologies like PSMA PET scans have made it possible to precisely identify metastatic sites early in their development. This has enabled targeted radiation to treat these sites directly—a strategy known as metastasis-directed therapy (MDT).

- MDT can be particularly effective for patients with oligometastatic disease.
- Precision radiation techniques such as Intensity Modulated Radiation Therapy (IMRT) and Stereotactic Body Radiotherapy (SBRT) are used to deliver highly focused doses to metastatic lesions while sparing surrounding healthy tissue.

3. Systemic Therapies

Systemic treatments remain essential for controlling widespread disease. They include the following:

- Androgen Deprivation Therapy (ADT): In its multivarious forms, ADT represents the historic foundation of systemic therapy for prostate cancer.
- Androgen Receptor Pathway Inhibitors: Drugs like enzalutamide (Xtandi), apalutamide (Erleada), abiraterone (Zytiga), and darolutamide (Nubeqa®) enhance ADT by blocking testosterone signaling more effectively than ADT alone.
- Chemotherapy: Docetaxel or cabazitaxel are often used in combination with hormone therapy.
- Radioligand Therapy: Agents like Xofigo (radium-223) and Pluvicto (lutetium-177 PSMA) deliver targeted radiation directly to cancer cells.
- Immunotherapy: Sipuleucel-T (Provenge) is an FDA-approved vaccine-based immunotherapy for advanced prostate cancer, often referred to "designer immunotherapy."
- Molecularly Targeted Therapies: Genomic profiling can identify actionable mutations for personalized treatments using PARP inhibitors or monoclonal antibodies.
- Precision Medicine: The role of state-of-the-art imaging technologies has revolutionized how metastatic prostate cancer is detected and managed.
  - PSMA PET Imaging provides unparalleled accuracy in identifying even small metastases.

- Combidex/USPIO Nanoparticle Imaging is used to detect the earliest microscopic lymph node involvement.

These tools allow clinicians to stratify patients into low-volume versus high-volume metastatic disease categories and tailor treatment plans accordingly.

Real-World Success Stories

At the Dattoli Cancer Center, these advanced concepts have been applied with remarkable success. Over the past two decades, many patients with advanced metastatic prostate cancer have achieved long-term complete remissions—many remaining cancer-free for well over 10 years—through aggressive yet precise protocols that are safe.

Key elements of our approach include:
- Dynamic Adaptive Radiation Therapy (DART), which is an extremely precise form of external beam radiation used to target both the prostate and regional lymph nodes.
- Metastasis-directed DART for skeletal or visceral metastases.
- Integration of systemic therapies such as ADT and androgen receptor inhibitors.
- Use of radioligand therapies (e.g., Xofigo, Pluvicto) and immunotherapies (e.g., Provenge).
- Molecular profiling to guide precision medicine strategies.

Toxicity profiles have been very mild, making these treatments both effective and well-tolerated by our patients, especially compared to chemotherapy.

The Path Forward

The treatment paradigm for metastatic prostate cancer has shifted dramatically from one of palliative care alone to one that embraces long-term curative potential.

A comprehensive strategy combining local therapies, metastasis-directed interventions, and systemic agents offers new hope for extending survival and improving quality of life.

For patients diagnosed with metastatic prostate cancer today—including both newly diagnosed patients and those who experience recurrence—there is no longer a single path forward but rather a spectrum of options tailored to individual needs and disease characteristics. By leveraging advances in imaging, precision medicine, and multidisciplinary care, we are entering an era where even advanced stages of this disease can be managed with much optimism about potential success in the near-term.

What is High Does Rate (HDR) Brachytherapy?

High Dose Rate (HDR) brachytherapy utilizes temporary prostate implants that utilize the isotope Iridium-192. This form of temporary brachytherapy is not new. It was first used in the early 1960s at Memorial Sloan-Kettering Cancer Center and has remained essentially unchanged since that time, with the exception of the current use of microprocessors and advanced imaging techniques.

The Iridium-192 isotope is encased inside a hollow plastic catheter less than 2 millimeters in diameter. Typically guided by ultrasound, these implants are inserted into the prostate and then removed, usually with two to four separate procedures spread over two to three days (though some centers are reporting short term results with a single, 1-day, high dose procedure). HDR sources deliver much higher doses of radiation in a much shorter period of time than permanent implants, with doses similar to EBRT.

Some limited studies have reported cure rates with the temporary HDR procedure that are comparable to those achieved by permanent implants. There is, however, far less long-term data regarding outcomes and side effects when compared to permanent implants. The HDR approach is not widely used for reasons of convenience and practicality. If performed in one setting, which would be optimal, the patient must remain in a semi-lithotomy position (legs pulled up) for upwards of 72 hours, with needles remaining in the prostate throughout this duration, with an indwelling urinary catheter and a drug administered to paralyze the bowel, to avoid any bowel movements.

Like external radiation, HDR is a form of fractionated radiation, which means radiation is administered only in intermittent doses. External radiation and HDR are often combined, with the Iridium-192 implant serving as a "boost" for an abbreviated course of external radiation.

Temporary implants usually require hospitalization and repeated implant procedures as opposed to the single permanent implant technique which can be done essentially on an out-patient basis. There may also be a greater risk of complications with HDR because of the extremely penetrating, high dose of radiation delivered by the Iridium-192 isotope (1000 to 2000 cGy in a matter of minutes).

A recent study from UCLA reported on intermediate risk patients treated with 6 fractions of HDR as monotherapy (without external radiation or hormonal therapy). The biochemical disease-free survival for these patients after 8 years of follow-up was 90%; however, biochemical failure was defined by these researchers according to less than stringent criteria (an increase of 2 ng/ml or more above the nadir PSA, that is, the lowest PSA reached following treatment). Only 68% of patients retained erectile function, and long-term genitourinary morbidity was more than 36.3%. (Patel S, et al, Brachytherapy, 2017 Mar - Apr;16(2):299-305).

An early study combining external radiation with HDR reported results with a 10-year follow-up. This study demonstrated a PSA progression-free survival rate of 90%, 87%, and 69% respectively for low, intermediate and high risk patients (Demanes DJ, et al, Int J Radiat Oncol Biol Phys. 2005 Apr 1;61(5):1306-16). Since the researchers on that study did not use a stringent PSA nadir value to determine treatment failure, the results are even less impressive. The study also showed that more than 7% of patients suffered from serious urinary morbidity (Grades 3 and 4), requiring some form of surgical intervention. Sexual potency was preserved in 67%, which also fails to measure up to the data reported on permanent brachytherapy, either alone or combined with external radiation.

A longer term German study also reported outcomes for HDR brachytherapy combined with EBRT. The results of that series showed biochemical freedom from disease for all patient risk groups combined, with 5, 10, and 15 year follow-up at 81.1%, 74%, and 67.8%, respectively (Galalae RM, et al, Brachytherapy, 2014 Mar-Apr;13(2):117-22). Those results are even less impressive because the definition of biochemical failure lacked the stringency of an absolute PSA nadir value. That study did not evaluate side effects.

A recent Australian study of HDR monotherapy with 10-year follow-up reported that for intermediate and high-risk patients, the biochemical disease-free survival rates were 86.9% and 56.1%, respectively. Patients with 3 high-risk factors had a biochemical survival of only 39.5%, and even that figure was inflated because these researchers did not employ a sufficiently stringent PSA nadir value to measure success. The study also reported that serious urethral strictures affected 13.6% of patients (Yaxley JW, et al, BJU Int, 2016 Sep 15).

Again, such results simply do not measure up to our published data with the combined treatment protocol of permanent brachytherapy and external radiation.

How are Permanent Seed Implants Planned and Performed?

At our institution, patients routinely undergo a pre-treatment staging and planning Color-Flow Power Doppler Ultrasound. That test, coupled with other staging studies such as MRI (Magnetic Resonance Imaging, preferably Multiparametric MRI and Dynamic Contrast Enhanced MRI—or DCE-MRI—which are utilized with PI-RADS Analysis and are superior to any other type of MRI currently available, including the spectroscopic MRI), ProstaScint® and 18F-FDG Fluoride/PET/CT Fusion studies, which allow us to visualize various physical aspects of the gland, such as its size, shape, and contour.

In addition, the use of encapsulated iron oxide nanoparticles or ultrasmall superparamagnetic iron oxide (USPIO), such as Feraheme, as MRI contrast agents is proving to be quite effective in identifying prostate cancer metastasis in the lymph nodes. At our institution, we have been involved in pioneering research with USPIO and now treating more advanced cases with lymph node involvement. (Dattoli MJ, et al, Efficacy of Feraheme as a Lymphatic Contrast Agent in Prostate Cancer, ASCO-GU Symposium, Feb 2018, and CIO Symposium on Clinical Interventional Oncology, Feb 2018).

All of these state-of-the-art tests also provide detailed information about the volume and location of the tumor (or tumors). With that information, we are able to determine exactly where the seeds should be placed. Additionally, this pre-treatment analysis may tell us if the pubic bones are going to pose any sort of obstacle when we perform the procedure. This is known as pubic arch interference, which we can usually circumvent by positioning the patient more advantageously. Later, in the operating room, the original plan can be modified since the gland position or contour changes when the pelvic muscles are relaxed under anesthesia. This is referred to as real time intraoperative planning to achieve optimal dosimetry.

Prior to the implant procedure, patients are asked not to eat after midnight the night before and the morning of the implant and are given pre-implant bowel cleansing instructions. A patient is admitted to the hospital as an outpatient for 23-hour observation. After admission, he is routinely given a prophylactic antibiotic. The patient is then brought into a dedicated brachytherapy surgical suite, and there undergoes an antiseptic skin cleansing. That is usually a Betadine solution applied to the perineal region. We are ready to proceed with the procedure after administering a local anesthetic (in most cases epidural or spinal anesthesia).

The procedure is done with the patient lying on his back, with his legs pulled up in what is called the extended lithotomy position. His legs are completely limp since a local anesthesia has been delivered. His feet are placed in comfortable booties and held in stirrups. Considerable time is spent ensuring that the patient is in the proper position and that the prostate is in the most desirable position. Then the implant procedure is performed using both ultrasound and fluoroscopic guidance.

The isotopes used for brachytherapy (except for Ir-192) don't deliver much radiation at a distance of a centimeter or centimeter and a half away from the gland, which is, for example, where the rectum and the bladder reside. The seeds are placed precisely at the site of the cancer within a margin of approximately 1 to 5 millimeters outside the prostate. By this means aided by Color-Flow Power Doppler Ultrasound visualizations, we can often deliver 2 to 5 times the dose with brachytherapy than we can with any other kind of radiation.

The dose rate is in the range of 20 cGy per hour with Palladium-103 compared to 5 to 10 cGy per hour with Iodine-125. A total dose of 12,500 cGy is typically delivered with Palladium-103 to full decay, while 14,400 cGy is typically delivered with Iodine-125. If we are supplementing the seed implant by preceding it with DART/IMRT, then the dose of the implant is reduced. With this combined or integrated approach, patients typically receive 4500 cGy of external radiation to a limited pelvic field, followed approximately two to eight weeks later by a Palladium-103 "boost." When combined with IMRT, the prescribed minimum Pd-103 dose to the prostate is 8000 to 9000 cGy with a suitable margin.

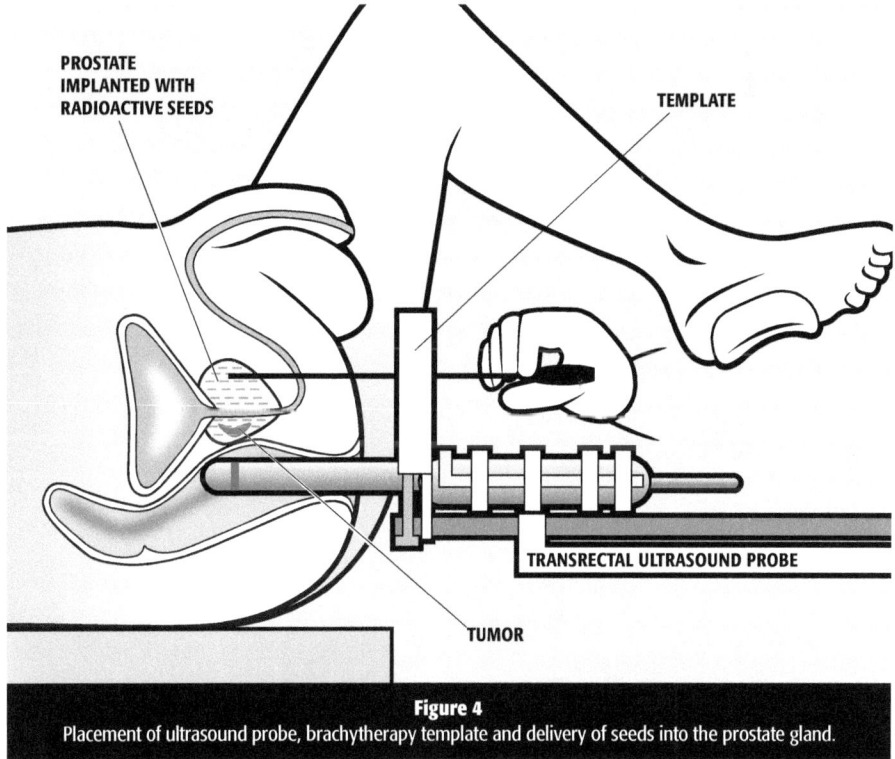

Figure 4
Placement of ultrasound probe, brachytherapy template and delivery of seeds into the prostate gland.

Seed implants are performed in a specially designed operating room (OR) where computers are accessible for intra-operative modifications. A well-trained OR staff is utilized for the procedure. Local anesthesia (spinal or epidural) is preferred. The advantage of a local anesthetic is that the patient feels little or no discomfort upon awakening, including that of a catheter, which is put into place during the implant procedure. Anti-inflammatory medications and antibiotics are routinely administered during and after the procedure (intraoperative and postoperative).

We maintain computers in the operating room since the contour of the prostate gland changes. This is an extremely common occurrence since this is the first time that we are looking at the prostate in a truly relaxed position without the pelvic muscles surrounding it being very tense. Because the patient has undergone a local anesthetic, he cannot tense up around the ultrasound probe which is placed in the rectum. Intraoperative modifications of the plan are made as necessary. Seed migration is not a problem since we use a special seed with very concave ends, and the tissue lodges in the edges, anchoring the seeds in place. We only use "free seeds" (rather than "stranded seeds") because this allows us maximal flexibility to make intraoperative changes as indicated and also allows us to place seeds outside the prostate. The tumor dose is escalated by locating the target with Color-Flow Power Doppler Ultrasound and by using seeds of different strengths to dose escalate the tumor and to dose demodulate critical structures such as the urethra, bladder and rectum.

The actual procedure, that is, the placement of the needles and insertion of the seeds, rarely takes longer than twenty-five minutes. The set-up time and preparation of the patient may take longer, and therefore, we generally book an hour and a half in the OR, because the patient has to be placed in the proper position and prepped for the procedure. It's very important to have the patient in a position that is identical to that of his pre-planning study in an attempt to duplicate the initial plan. When performing the procedure, special crisscross anchoring needles are used to maximally immobilize the prostate gland. These two crisscross needles are inserted transperineally, obliquely into the prostate, using finger and fluoroscopic guidance. These needles are left in place during the procedure to anchor the prostate in place, preventing any movement during the procedure.

Seeds are commonly placed in extraprostatic positions to further target the tumor, which may be microscopically escaping from the gland (see Color Image 5). This technique of placing seeds 1 to 5 millimeters *outside* the gland also allows for reduction of the urethral dose. This is important since the main side effect of brachytherapy is temporary urethritis. Additionally, the extraprostatic technique allows for treating patients who have had prior TURPs with a far reduced incontinence rate (see below, "How are Implants Modified for Patients with Prior TURPs?").

After the procedure, the patient is transferred to a private room and monitored closely throughout his stay. Although many brachytherapists discharge their patients soon after the implant is complete, at our institution the patient is kept overnight. The indwelling catheter is left in place for a minimum of 12 hours and dislodges any tissue, clots or debris that could present future problems (urinary blockage). The catheter is removed only when upon inspection the urine is perfectly clear. Usually, the catheter is kept in place until three o'clock in the morning. That saves a lot of grief for the patient and for the doctors and nurses by eliminating those calls that might come late at night when the patient potentially has some blockage. By keeping the catheter in and irrigating the bladder, we have eliminated this problem.

For the most part, patients have a very easy time with seed implants. The most common question asked after the procedure is, "When are you going to start?" Many are still waiting for the procedure to begin when they realize it has already taken place. Patients rarely complain of specific pains in the perineal region, that area where the seeds are implanted between the scrotal sac and the anus. The only discomfort that a patient may have is more likely to be a consequence of the catheter later in the day or evening when the regional anesthetic has worn off. That may be felt more than the tiny needles which are utilized to insert the seeds.

The patient is discharged the morning following the procedure, usually in excellent spirits and ready to return home whether far away or locally. Prior to his leaving our center, special stereo-shift x-rays and helical CT scans are taken to count seeds and to ensure there are no potential complications (for example, abscess formation or hematomas from bleeding, though these are uncommon). Patients will then return for a comprehensive evaluation at approximately 3 months, and then 6 to 12 months thereafter. Ultimately, we request that patients return annually for monitoring.

Which Patients are Eligible for Brachytherapy?

Most patients can safely tolerate the implant procedure as it is minimally invasive and requires only light anesthesia. Men with a history of heart disease or stroke are usually given a thorough medical evaluation, including a cardiac stress test, before proceeding with seed implantation.

If you are a candidate for surgery, you are almost surely also a candidate for seed implants, as both treatments are most effective with early stage cancers. In addition, many men who would not be candidates for surgery—those patients over the age of 70, or those men with other health conditions that rule out major surgery—may qualify as candidates for seeding, which is a much less invasive procedure than radical prostatectomy. As we will see, recent data indicates that patients with high risk features are more likely to have a successful outcome with brachytherapy combined with external radiation (preferably DART/4D IG-IMRT) than would be expected with surgery.

The most important factor in determining a patient's eligibility for seeding is how far the cancer has spread. If the cancer is localized, that is, confined to the prostate gland, then it is more likely to be curable, with either surgery or seeding. Once the cancer has spread outside the prostate, it is not curable by implantation alone, because the seed implants do not radiate enough area around the prostate to destroy any cancer that may have spread outside the prostate. These patients are similarly not candidates for radical prostatectomy.

Patients with stage T1 are most likely to have cancer that is confined to the prostate, and therefore, curable with seed implantation alone. With that said, having treated over the years thousands of low risk patients with seeds alone, and followed them for 10 to 20 years, we have witnessed an increased failure rate (as many as 50% of these patients typically after 10 years) when compared to low risk or even intermediate risk patients who were treated with a combination of seeds and external beam radiation. For this reason, we encourage combined treatment even for low risk patients since the side effect profile is the same or even slightly reduced with the combined approach. The last telephone call we ever want to make to a patient is to tell him that his PSA is rising. We believe the multi-modality approach improves survival rates. By combining external beam radiation and seeds, the cancer is being exposed to two different forms of radiation and is more likely to be eradicated.

Patients with locally advanced disease may be treated either with external radiation or with a combination of seed implants and external radiation (preferably DART/4D IG-IMRT). These patients include those with one or more of the following risk factors: stage equal to or greater than T2b, a Gleason score greater than or equal to 7, a PSA greater than 10, an elevated PAP, or radiographic evidence of extraprostatic extension (as indicated by Color-Flow Power Doppler Ultrasound, Multiparametric MRI, Dynamic Contrast Enhanced MRI, endorectal MRI, MRSI, ProstaScint® / CT Fusion, 18F-FDG Fluoride PET/CT Fusion, and other advanced imaging techniques).

Seed implants should only be considered by patients who are young enough and healthy enough to live long enough to benefit from being cured. Excellent candidates are men from their forties to their seventies, with localized prostate cancer. Some men in their eighties who are in good health may also benefit from implantation, and an increasing number of men in their thirties are now being treated with these methods. After all, younger patients stand to benefit most from therapies that will preserve their quality of life, including continence and erectile function.

Patients who have had a portion of their prostate removed with a previous TURP may be at increased risk for urinary incontinence after seeding, in which case, special modifications of seed placement may be necessary when possible (peripheral seed loading and especially sparing the external sphincter). Patients with enlarged prostates and those men who have difficulty with urination prior to treatment may have more severe urinary problems after implantation. Treatment is typically limited to men with prostates less than 60 cubic centimeters volume. For patients with enlarged prostates, two or three months of hormonal therapy before implantation may be prescribed in order to shrink the gland. Larger glands may also be implanted based on other anatomical considerations.

What are the Most Common Myths About Brachytherapy?

Myth # 1: "Your tumor is too aggressive to be effectively treated by brachytherapy." This assertion is often made by urologists, who suggest that a high PSA and/or a high Gleason score disqualifies patients for seed implants. In fact, the published results of combined brachytherapy and external beam radiation with intermediate and high risk patients are superior to surgical results even at the leading surgical centers.

Myth # 2: "Your prostate gland is too small for brachytherapy." Patients with smaller glands may hear this from their urologists, but the statement is absolutely false. Brachytherapy can treat smaller glands very effectively, specifically, by putting seeds outside the prostate gland (the technique known as "extraprostatic seed placement"). By placing the seeds in this fashion, the dose to the urethra can actually be decreased while the target area receives an effective, cancericidal dose.

Myth # 3: "Your prostate gland is too large for brachytherapy." This is another urological myth. By extending the lithotomy position, which is the position with the legs up in the air, and/or by using steering needles, problems with pubic arch interference can be circumvented. In this way, seed implants can be utilized with patients who have larger prostates. In addition, larger glands can often be downsized with hormonal therapy.

Myth # 4: "Once you've had brachytherapy, you've burned your bridges. Surgery cannot be performed after implantation, and you won't have any other salvage options if the seeds fail." In fact, an expert surgeon will be able to remove the prostate after seed implantation. However, the patient may choose one of a number of other options. Since he chose not to have surgery in the first place, he may choose re-seeding, with or without 4-Dimensional Image Guided IMRT with DART. At our center, we do use another isotope, because clearly if the cancer failed the first isotope, we want to give it something else that it's not acclimated to. So if a patient was seeded with Iodine-125, he may have an improved outcome with Palladium-103. The patient can also choose cryosurgery as a salvage therapy, or biothermy, which combines cryosurgery and hyperthermia. High Intensity Frequency Ultrasound would be another option, and researchers are working on vaccines for which there are clinical trials underway.

Myth # 5: "You are a young patient, and therefore, radiation may increase your risk of developing a secondary cancer." There is a great deal of data showing this assertion to be false. Recent studies have reported that contemporary radiation does not increase the risk of future colo-rectal cancer (Kendall, et al, *Int. J Rad Onc,* Vol 65, No 3, 2006, and Gotman, et al, *Int. J Rad Onc,* Vol 66, No 1, 2006). This myth is based on old data when radiation oncologists were treating with external beams and large-field boxes, and they were basically treating normal tissue in addition to the prostate or lymph nodes in order to deliver radiation to those structures. The accuracy of our current state-of-the-art technology eliminates the risk of developing secondary cancers after brachytherapy and 4D IG-IMRT with DART.

Myth # 6: "You are too young to have brachytherapy." This is yet another falsehood. In this regard, outstanding biochemical outcomes have been reported for younger patients and this group has the most to gain (reduced risk of urinary incontinence and/or erectile dysfunction). Of the numerous studies published by Blasko (2005), Kwok (2002), Kollmeir (2003), Dattoli (2009), all have mean and median follow-up which is equal to or longer than the surgical series published in the PSA era.

Myth # 7: "You are too old to have brachytherapy." The truth is that older patients tolerate brachytherapy as well as younger patients. Many patients as well as doctors are not aware of the fact that life expectancy is quite long and becoming longer with each passing year. As such, more and more older patients can and should be treated, especially with non-invasive treatments such as brachytherapy and other sophisticated forms of radiation.

Myth # 8: "If you had a prior TURP (transurethral resection of the prostate), you are not a candidate for brachytherapy." Many urologists suggest that a prior TURP is a contraindication for seed implants, but that is simply not the case. The Dattoli team has published extensively on this subject, showing that it can be done, but the patient with a prior TURP must be carefully evaluated. Each patient is different. There has to be enough tissue to put the seeds into the gland. If the TURP was a "Roto-Rooter" and removed too much tissue, there may not be enough tissue left to anchor the seeds. In addition, special efforts must be made to avoid incontinence. Another issue is avoiding a hot apex, which is the bottom of the gland. A patient who has had a TURP has already had his internal sphincter removed, and so we have to be concerned about his external sphincter, his lower sphincter. We have learned that external radiation (4D IG-IMRT with DART), combined with brachytherapy, reduces the risk of problems with these patients (see "How are Implants Modified for Patients with Prior TURPs?").

In February 2021, the Dattoli Team presented a paper for the American Society of Clinical Oncology (ASCO), Genitourinary Symposium. The subject of the abstract was the safety of photoselective vaporization of the prostate in the contact of the DART and brachytherapy combined protocol—Dattoli M.J. et al, Risk of urinary morbidity associated with photoselective vaporization of the prostate (PVP) in prostate cancer patients undergoing a combined radiotherapy regimen consisting of dynamic adaptive radiotherapy (DART) and brachytherapy boost—reprinted as an Interactive Poster Presentation by the International Journal Hem-Onc, retrieved December, 2021—https://www.hem-onc.org/poster-05-dattoli.

With regard to this TURP issue, please note: With modern peripheral seed placement where epithelial (TURP) defect is limited to ≤110% of the minimum peripheral dose, results in reduced incontinence/leakage are similar to that of non-TURP patients, taking into account the following considerations:

- The gland must have sufficient tissue remaining to anchor seeds.
- Case selection is paramount to avoid overly extensive TURP.
- Avoidance of hot apex and supplemental IMRT may even further reduce risks of urinary incontinence/leakage.

Myth # 9: "You are too overweight to have brachytherapy." Contrary to this notion, the reality is that brachytherapy patients who are overweight enjoy a higher rate of success with seed implants than with surgery. In fact, brachytherapy is the most preferred treatment for obese patients. A high body mass index (BMI) translates into increased hospital stays after surgery. Comparing surgery and brachytherapy in terms of biochemical failure with high BMI patients, as the body mass index goes up, the surgical relapse rate goes up as well, while brachytherapy achieves excellent results with these patients.

Myth # 10: "You have an elevated AUA score and that precludes you from having brachytherapy." The AUA score provides a profile of urinary and rectal symptoms. An elevated AUA score in many cases is not a contraindication for seed implants. Even patients with voiding symptoms can tolerate brachytherapy. This may be because doctors have learned how to micro-manage these symptoms. There have been a number of studies investigating long term urinary morbidity after seed implantation. One study demonstrated that "patients who presented with marked urinary symptoms prior to brachytherapy had the most significant improvement in symptoms and quality of life after brachytherapy at a median follow-up of 31 months" (Stone et al, *J. Brachy. Int.,* Vol 2, 2003). Another recent study showed there was no significant difference in the overall long-term urinary and quality of life (QoL) scores when brachytherapy patients were compared to a control group (Merrick et al, *IJROBP*, Vol 56, 2003).

When is Hormonal Therapy used in Conjunction with Seeding and External Radiation?

Hormonal therapy (also known as Androgen Deprivation Therapy, or ADT) is typically optional at our institution for patients having intermediate risk features but encouraged for patients having high risk features. Simply put, certain hormones have the ability to temporarily halt or slow the growth of prostate cancer, as well as to shrink the overall size of the gland (as much as 50%). Men with enlarged prostates can benefit by reducing the size of the prostate gland, making it a smaller target for radiation treatment.

With the low-risk or mildly aggressive cancers, unless the size of the gland is markedly large, we don't normally give the conventional hormonal therapy (combined hormonal blockade using an androgen and an LHRH agonist, such as Lupron®, Eligard®, Zoladex® or Trelstar®), since this form of therapy may result in untoward side effects such as erectile dysfunction, hot flashes and potential weakness. We often prescribe a milder, modified version of hormones (e.g. oral anti-androgens), something that is just enough to arrest the cancer and allow the patient to make a more relaxed decision about treatment, without the rush or urgency that are often associated with it.

What is Neoadjuvant Hormonal Therapy?

Neoadjuvant Hormonal Therapy employs hormonal agents before primary curative therapies such as radiotherapy, radical surgery (prostatectomy), and cryosurgery. The primary goal of neoadjuvant therapy is to enhance the effectiveness of the primary therapy by shrinking the tumor before treatment.

A number of studies have shown improved results at local control of the disease and survival for higher risk patients when hormonal therapy is administered prior to and following external beam radiation therapy and brachytherapy. The landmark study in this area was a European clinical trial, EORTC 22863 (Eur Urol. 1998 Dec; 35 Suppl S1:23-26.). That was the first study to demonstrate an overall survival benefit of radiation therapy combined with hormones versus radiation alone.

Another clinical trial, RTOG 9202, published by the Radiation Therapy Oncology

Group, showed that adjuvant ADT before, during and 24 months after RT showed a significant survival advantage for patients with Gleason scores 8 to 10 (Hanks et al, J Clin Oncol. 2003 Nov 1;21(21):3972-8). The dose of radiation utilized in these early clinical trials was low compared to our current dosimetry protocols with DART and brachytherapy.

A large multi-institutional study in 2016 showed that men with metastatic prostate cancer had significantly improved survival when treated with ADT in addition to radiation therapy over radiotherapy alone (Improved Survival With Prostate Radiation in Addition to Androgen Deprivation Therapy for Men With Newly Diagnosed Metastatic Prostate Cancer, Rusthoven CG, et al, J Clin Oncol. 2016 Aug 20;34(24):2835-42).

Another large multi-institutional study in 2017 reported the men with recurrent prostate cancer treated with radiotherapy and 24 months of ADT had "significantly higher rates of long-term overall survival and lower incidences of metastatic prostate cancer and death from prostate cancer" than patients treated with radiation alone (Radiation with or without Antiandrogen Therapy in Recurrent Prostate Cancer, Shipley WJ, et al, N Engl J Med. 2017 Feb 2;376(5):417-428).

Though not definitive, the results of these studies and others are seen as encouraging by many researchers. Many of us believe that hormonal therapy and radiation have a synergistic effect in eradicating the cancer, especially in high-risk patients. At the same time, it should be noted that no advantage has been found for neoadjuvant ADT given with radiation for low-risk patients.

Recent studies of combined treatment modalities have also helped to determine our clinical protocol for combining ADT with brachytherapy, Dynamic Adaptive Radiation Therapy (DART), and all modalities associated with 4-Dimensional Image Guided Intensity Modulated Radiation Therapy (4D IG-IMRT). For additional information and guidance with regard to ADT and radiotherapy, readers are referred to our companion Prostate Cancer Essentials booklet, *Hormonal Therapy for Prostate Cancer: The Benefits and Risks*.

What are the Possible Side Effects of Seed Implantation?

Seed implantation involves significantly less risk of long-term complications compared with surgery or conventional EBRT. Side effects with implants are usually mild and reversible. The most common organ system involved with temporary side effects from seed implants is the urinary tract, and this is because the prostate is nestled beneath the bladder and has the urethra running through it. Following implantation, most patients experience increased urinary frequency and urgency, a weakened stream, and occasionally, urinary burning. Fortunately, these symptoms are temporary and resolve as the radioactivity of the seeds dissipates over time.

With palladium implants, the 17-day half-life typically causes about two and a half to four months of some type of urinary symptomatology. With the 60-day half-life of iodine implants, urinary symptoms may persist for ten to twelve months. During this period, we do our best to micromanage these urinary symptoms with a variety of medications. The symptoms are in no way debilitating, but rather more of a nuisance, and patients are encouraged to continue their normal level of activity.

While side effects with implantation are usually temporary, there is some risk of more serious, permanent complications, including urinary incontinence (in less than 1% of patients) and erectile dysfunction. When they do occur, such side effects usually appear 6 to 24 months after treatment. As mentioned, patients who have previously undergone TURPs are at higher risk for developing incontinence. Incontinence is a very rare complication associated with implantation therapy in general for patients without TURPs—less than 1% in virtually all studies. But patients with prior TURPs are more likely to develop urinary incontinence, up to 50% according to some researchers. However, brachytherapists who modify their implants and make adjustments for patients with TURPs have reported incontinence in less than 3% of patients (see below, "How are Implants Modified for Patients with Prior TURPs?").

Another potential side effect with seeds is irritation to the rectum, although this is uncommon. In our experience with the procedure, we haven't had any patients who have had to have a colostomy or who have a persistent rectal ulceration; nor have we had any patients who required urinary diversion because of damage to the urethra. It appears that while the urethra tends to play an important role with seeding in terms of the side effect profile, it generally is able to withstand the dose, and once the radiation isotopes decay, the side effects disappear.

There are many factors that may influence the duration of urinary symptoms, including prostatitis, enlarged prostates, dietary intake, and non-compliance with prescribed medications. These are routinely managed as indicated. *It should be also noted that patients who have received IMRT prior to brachytherapy, do not experience any significant increase in the temporary side effects associated with implantation* (see, "What is Intensity Modulated Radiation Therapy?").

At our institution, after a patient is discharged following brachytherapy, a number of medications are commonly prescribed. These include the following:

> ➢ An anti-inflammatory to help reduce swelling of the prostate. Typically, a steroid anti-inflammatory will be used for several days, and thereafter a non-steroidal anti-inflammatory such as ibuprofen.

- An over-the-counter medication like Pepcid® AC may be used with the anti-inflammatory to prevent stomach upset.
- An antibiotic is routinely prescribed to prevent infection of the prostate.
- An alpha-blocker such as Flomax®, Uroxotral®, Hytrin® or Cardura® is prescribed to aid the flow of urination. This is the most important medication for the treatment of urinary symptoms. Patients usually continue using an alpha-blocker for several weeks to several months, depending on the duration of symptoms. It should also be noted there have been studies showing quinazoline-based alpha blockers (Hytrin®, Cardura®, and Uroxotrol®), actually induce prostate cancer cell death (apoptosis).
- Hydrocortisone suppositories are used as a preventative medication to address any rectal irritation that may result from the ultrasound rectal probe used during the seeding procedure, or from irritation caused by the radiation, or from pre-existing hemorrhoids.
- Over-the-counter medications such as Azo Standard® or Azo Cranberry®, sodium bicarbonate tablets, or Prelief® may be used to help with any urinary burning or discomfort.
- Over-the-counter preparations such as Metamucil or Citracel may be used for constipation or looseness of the bowels.

It should also be noted that radiation patients are advised to avoid all antioxidant supplements such as Vitamins A, C, E, beta carotene and selenium, as these may have an opposing action to the radiation treatment.

What is the Risk of Erectile Dysfunction After Seed Implantation?

Generally speaking, patients having prostate brachytherapy will have erectile dysfunction in about 15% to 20% of cases, although some institutions are reporting higher rates of incidence. Brachytherapy does not appear to produce the steady decline of potency that we have seen with full course external beam radiation through the years. Rather, we have noted not only a leveling off of the potency rate over time after implantation, but even a gradual improvement over time. Essentially, where you are at two to three years after treatment is where you will likely be as far as erectile function, taking into account that patients are getting older and may be taking hypertensive medications, diabetic medications or have other medical problems which could interfere with erectile function over time. Smoking and obesity are also significant causal factors for erectile dysfunction. It should be noted that a diminished ejaculate with a clearer consistency, which may occur after seed implantation, should not be confused with having serious erectile dysfunction, which is the loss of ability to produce and/or sustain an erection sufficient for intercourse.

For those men who lose potency, Viagra® (sildenafil), intracavernosal paparavine, and Prostaglandin E1 injections are very effective. Viagra® has altered the clinical situation considerably. According to one study, for men who are potent at the time of treatment, 92% of patients having seed implants (with or without supplemental external radiation) will maintain erectile function potency. Two additional oral erectile aids, Levitra® (Vardenafil) and Cialis® (Tadalafil) are also available.

It should also be noted that the risk of erectile dysfunction may be reduced with Palladium-103 because of one of its unique physical properties. The *radial dose fall-off,* that is, the amount of radiation actually delivered at any distance from the Pd-103 seed, is less with palladium than with any other isotope. Therefore, palladium is less likely to over-radiate the neurovascular bundles or proximal penile tissues, both of which affect the ability to have and maintain an erection. Moreover, the dose to the penile bulb approaches nil using 4D IG-IMRT with DART (compared with 40% to 50% with standard IMRT).

How Do Seed Implants Affect Sexual Activity?

There are no formal restrictions on sexual activity after seed implantation. A patient can resume sexual activities immediately. Some men may not wish to engage in sex right away as the area may be somewhat irritated. As a safety precaution, patients receiving Pd-103 seeds are advised to utilize a condom for a three week period after implantation, so as to avoid the unlikely possibility of ejaculating a seed into his partner. That precaution is extended for patients receiving I-125 seeds because of their longer half-life.

For the majority of patients who retain potency, the major change that we see after implantation is the diminution in the volume of the ejaculate. Shortly after the implant, there may also be a discoloring or a different consistency to the ejaculate. Typically it's described as being clearer and thinner, but the majority of patients have little problem with that as long as they're able to maintain an erection and achieve orgasm.

A patient can have normal sperm after implantation. The testicles are a separate organ from the prostate *per se,* and while there may be a short period of oligospermia (a decrease in the sperm count), a patient very well may have a return of sperm. Although there is little chance that radiation will affect the sperm, attempts to impregnate should be avoided for at least six months. Because of the diminished ejaculate, and the change in milieu that the sperm will encounter, the chance of successful impregnation is probably greatly reduced, though several of our patients have successfully conceived. We counsel our patients that they need to be careful and should not consider themselves to be sterile because of the procedure. At the same time, men wanting to father children should always consider banking sperm before implantation.

What Precautions Should Patients Exercise After the Implant Procedure?

After implantation, patients are advised for the first month not to hold children less than two years of age for extended periods—for hours in a day or for consecutive days. This applies only to Palladium-103 implants, because that isotope has a short half-life and delivers its dose relatively quickly. With Iodine-125 implants, a longer period of restraint needs to be exercised. These restrictions do not mean having no contact. Even during the period immediately after the implant, a patient can have casual contact with children less than two years old. It's perfectly safe for a seeding patient to hold a child on his lap for brief periods.

How are Implants Modified for Patients with Prior TURPs?

A *transurethral resection of the prostate*, or TURP, is a surgical procedure used to remove tissue obstructing the urethra in patients with enlarged prostates due to *benign prostatic hyperplasia* (BPH). If a patient has had a TURP, the seed implant procedure has to be mapped out very carefully, and the seeds need to be distributed differently in that particular patient. They have to be positioned in a way that avoids the TURP itself; otherwise, they may be deposited into an empty prostatic cavity and eventually be urinated out. Misplaced seeds may cause potential damage in that way. With these patients, we use a seed loading pattern that is very peripheral to the gland, placing seeds in extraprostatic positions and taking care to avoid the remaining external sphincter.

The reason that incontinence risks may be high in these patients is because a TURP typically removes the superior internal sphincter, leaving the patient with only the lower sphincter. The high doses of implant radiation may impair that sphincter's ability to work normally. Another factor to consider is how large the TURP is compared to the size of the prostate. There must be enough prostate tissue around the TURP to anchor the seeds; if the TURP is excessive, there may not be enough tissue for the seeds to adhere. That might be a contraindication to seed implantation, though it's rare in our practice that a prior TURP would prevent a patient from being seeded.

For men who have been treated for BPH with photoselective vaporization of the prostate (PVP) rather than TURP, we have shown that there is little risk of serious urinary symptoms following the combined protocol of DART and brachytherapy. PVP techniques include both Green Laser and Olympus Plasma Button (Dattoli MJ, et al, (Risk of urinary morbidity associated with photoselective vaporization of the prostate (PVP) in prostate cancer patients undergoing a combined radiotherapy regimen consisting of dynamic adaptive radiotherapy (DART and brachytherapy boost; American Society of Clinical Oncology (ASCO), Genitourinary Symposium, February, 2021).

What are the Advantages of Palladium-103 Over Iodine-125?

The choice of palladium versus iodine is typically based on physician preference, although it is sometimes decided by the patient. While there is some controversy regarding which is superior, at our institution with a large brachytherapy practice, palladium is preferred and its advantages have been confirmed.

Radiobiological considerations suggest that palladium would be more effective against rapidly growing, more aggressive cancers (those with higher Gleason scores) as well as low-grade prostate malignancies. While there have been no definitive (prospective, randomized) human clinical trials to date comparing tumor-control rates with Pd-103 and I-125, studies have reported a lower complication rate for Pd-103, as well as a more precipitous fall in PSA levels and reduced incidence of benign PSA "bounce" (see below, "What is PSA Bounce?"). As mentioned, the duration of temporary side effects is shorter with palladium because of its shorter half-life.

What are the Advantages of Combining Seed Implants with External Radiation Therapy?

Over the past decade we have seen the pendulum swing dramatically from patients in the past who strongly desired to undergo seed implantations alone to more recent patients who desire the combination method of IMRT or 4 Dimensional Image-Guided Radiation Therapy (4D-IGRT) and brachytherapy. This trend is due to a number of factors. These days many patients do extensive research and find that there is always a real risk of having extraprostatic disease extension, which is more effectively treated by integrating seed implants with external radiation therapy (IMRT or 4D-IGRT). Many patients now understand that with IMRT (and especially 4D IG-IMRT with DART) they are afforded the added security of covering possible extraprostatic extension while experiencing little to no additional side effects.

Why Should Seed Implants Be Done After External Radiation?

When external radiation is combined with brachytherapy, the sequence is typically EBRT (preferably 4D IG-IMRT) followed by an implant boost, with the doses of each modality moderated to achieve optimal coverage while at the same time limiting rectal, bladder and urethral doses. The history of the combined approach suggests there may be considerable reason for concern that reversing the sequence (implant first followed by external radiation) may increase the risk of rectal complications, in part because there is a significant interval when patients are receiving simultaneous implant and external radiation.

We have learned that by targeting the tumor and its extensions first with 4D IG-IMRT, with or without hormonal therapy, the seeding procedure is more effective and serves as a boost, while not leaving the migrating cells in the regions outside of the prostate untreated. The surrounding pelvic field is essentially sterilized and cancers are rendered nonviable when IMRT is used before the seed implantation. Some doctors who have treated in the reverse order, implanting seeds before administering external radiation, have reported higher rates of rectal injury. There is also concern that implanting seeds first in intermediate or high grade cancers may spread cancer into the bloodstream. This potential threat is eliminated with the implant-boost approach, because the external radiation has sterilized the peripheral field prior to the insertion of implant needles.

As noted, traditionally, patients at the Dattoli Cancer Center are treated to an initial dose level of approximately 4500 cGy prior to interstitial brachytherapy. This dose level typically covers not only the prostate, but also potentially surrounding target tissues (including, but not limited to, seminal vesicles, periprostatic lymph nodes, obturator lymph nodes, internal iliac lymph nodes, and even common iliac and para-aortic nodes per individual case as indicated).

A 4100 cGy dose was initially chosen since early physics and radiobiologic evaluations performed by physicists at Memorial Sloan Kettering (MSKCC), especially Dr. Lowell Anderson, suggested that this dose given along with an attenuated dose of Palladium-103 of 8000-9000 cGy would not exceed rectal, urethral or bladder tolerances. The 4100 cGy dose has since been increased to 4500 cGy using sophisticated IMRT technologies.

Bear in mind that in the latter 1980's, no one knew the correct doses when combining EBRT + Pd-103. At that time, the Pd-103 isotope was relatively new and

Dr. Anderson was instrumental in characterizing the physical parameters and laid the groundwork for clinical models.

During that time, Dr. Dattoli worked closely with Dr. Anderson and other physicists at MSKCC and adopted these dose parameters, and since then, he has never had an incidence of rectal fistula or urethral-rectal fistula. The dose of 4500 cGy, however, is insufficient in most cases to eradicate microscopic, and especially potentially macroscopic cancer cells, at a distance from the prostate gland. For this reason, following the implant procedure, our physics/dosimetry staff then generates precise isodose curves emanating from the seed implant (both inside and outside the gland).

The dose projected by the seeds to a given distance from the prostate can then be precisely calculated up to the point of near complete decay of the palladium-103 at the three month mark after seeding. For this reason, most patients return approximately three months after seeding (at the point of near decay of the isotope) to receive a small number of additional 4D IG-IMRT treatments to peripheral target tissue sites while blocking the prostate, bladder, rectum, and proximal penile tissues.

The individualization of the dose is multifactorial which may include taking into account the size of the gland, stage, size of tumor(s), location of tumor(s), Gleason score, PSA, PAP, prior TURP/TUIP, etc. The optimal dose to target points at distance from the gland, and the subsequent physics analysis will determine the number of treatments necessary to achieve the desired dose. It is to be noted that this methodology has been in place since the mid-1990's, although, is now more liberally utilized with IMRT in view of the safety associated with dose escalation using this newer modality.

What are the Results of the Dattoli Combined Radiotherapy Protocol?

The treatment protocol combining brachytherapy with DART has been perfected by Dr. Dattoli and his colleagues, over a 20-year period, and has produced **the longest and best published cure rate** in all the medical literature. With our current combination protocol, patients having low risk disease enjoy a greater than 95% biochemical success rate while, thanks to our advanced DART technology, we are now seeing even those patients having intermediate to high-risk disease achieving an approximate 90% cure rate with remarkably few, temporary side effects. Having treated patients with lymph node cancer and even bone metastases successfully, we are moving up the ladder in terms of the stage of the disease that can be conquered.

Our results have improved each year with refinements in technique and technology. As of 2010, our published data (*Journal of Oncology*, August, 2010) on patients with higher risk disease reported an 82% biochemical success rate with a follow up of 16 years.

Those results have continued to improve in recent years. It is important to note that those patients were treated between 1992 and 1997 with combination of Palladium-103 brachytherapy and 3D Conformal Radiation Therapy, which during that decade was the most sophisticated form of external radiation therapy available. We have come a long way since that time with our current state-of-the-art DART capabilities and constantly improving seed implantation methods, translating into even more successful results.

The data that we published for higher risk patients is especially important because the vast majority of those patients treated in our 16-year series were considered incurable using any other treatment method, especially radical prostatectomy. To date, no other practitioners in the world have reported results as successful as our long-term series with higher risk patients. As mentioned, the biochemical cure rate for low risk patients in our practice is typically greater than 95%, which is comparable or superior to the results achieved by the other leading brachytherapy teams. When treating intermediate and high risk disease, we simply have no peers.

Yet as impressive as the published results are, they do not reflect the effectiveness of our current technologies and skills. As we continue to follow our patients, we believe our cure rates to be even higher, given the much higher doses that can be delivered with DART and the far greater accuracy, **which now enables us to most effectively eradicate the cancer while minimizing side effects—and we accomplish this one patient at a time.**

At our center, patients credit the Dattoli Team's combination therapy program for significantly reducing the chance of long-term side effects that most other treatment options pose, such as incontinence (loss of bladder control), and sexual impotence (loss of erectile function). Other more invasive surgical procedures such as radical prostatectomy have a higher risk of treatment failure and potential complications, as well as a considerably longer period of recovery. Likewise, high-dose rate radiation therapies in various forms pose a much higher risk of treatment failure and potential adverse side effects.

A recent study by the Dana Farber Cancer Center, Brigham & Women's Hospital and Harvard Medical School cited two groundbreaking studies by Dr. Dattoli utilizing his treatment protocol that combines external radiation therapy (EBRT) with a brachytherapy boost. The Dana Farber study lamented the decline of brachytherapy in recent years because the data shows that seed implantation combined with external beam radiotherapy is by far the most effective treatment for prostate cancer (Orio PF, et al., The decreased use of brachytherapy boost for intermediate and high-risk prostate cancer despite evidence supporting its effectiveness, Brachytherapy 15(6) June 2016).

Brachytherapy has become something of a 'lost art' because many radiation oncologists can make more money by utilizing 15 to 20 additional EBRT treatment sessions without the seed implant boost. These unscrupulous physicians are cashing in on Medicare and insurance reimbursements rather than providing their patients with the highest quality of care. Brachytherapy combined with EBRT has been shown to be more cost effective for patients and is also far more effective at eradicating prostate cancer.

Unfortunately, there are many radiation oncologists who have joined with urologists in profit-making ventures offering a range of lucrative treatments options from robotic radical surgery to high dose, hypofractionated Intensity Modulated Radiation Therapy (IMRT). Our advice is 'buyer beware,' with each patient now a potential buyer. We strongly encourage all patients to become informed and to make decisions about their treatment by taking into account the evidence-based data for each currently available treatment option.

What is a PSA Bounce?

About 30% to 40% of patients undergoing seed implantation experience a temporary rise in PSA after an initial decline in their PSA level following treatment. This phenomenon is known as a PSA bounce or flare. It generally occurs approximately 18–24 months after treatment and is not caused by a recurrence of cancer, but rather by radiation-induced prostatitis (inflammation of the prostate) with subsequent systemic release of PSA. These patients are still considered disease-free. The rise in PSA may be 0.1 or higher and can sometimes last many months, but it is usually of short duration. Studies have shown that the PSA bounce is more common with younger patients, those who receive higher implant doses, and those with larger prostate glands.

One 40-year-old patient saw his PSA rise to 28.6 two years after brachytherapy. This unusually large bounce caused him considerable distress and uncertainty. Repeat staging studies were negative, although urologists wanted to remove his prostate gland. The patient, fortunately, did not have his gland removed and his PSA steadily declined. His most recent PSA reading at ten years was 0.001.

What Are RapidArc™, Volumetric Modulated Arc Therapy (VMAT), and the TrueBeam™ System?

According to the manufacturer, Varian Medical Systems, RapidArc™ is a technological innovation that delivers a complete IMRT treatment with a single rotation of the linear accelerator delivery system around the patient. This technology is known as Volumetric Modulated Arc Therapy or Rotational Radiotherapy, and the main advantage touted by the manufacturer is that treatment time may be 2 to 10 times faster than earlier generations of IMRT systems, including DART. The accelerated treatment time (under 3 minutes) would enable a cancer center using this technology to treat many more patients; however, it should be noted that the safety and efficacy of this approach have not been demonstrated. RapidArc™ has been licensed by the FDA and is being aggressively marketed, but it is still entirely experimental. There are no studies demonstrating the long term safety of such rapid, extremely high dose rate delivery. We are concerned that RapidArc™ may be shown to damage healthy tissue and cause secondary cancers and late side effects in the years following treatment.

In order to incorporate RapidArc™, a fully realized IMRT system must be in place along with a patient information management system known as Aria™. RapidArc™ is a very costly approach that initially sounds promising, but the reality is that with arc therapy, the integral dose will be higher with a continuous open beam (arc) of radiation directed at the patient (see "Radiotherapy Treatment Plans With RapidArc for Prostate Cancer Involving Seminal Vesicles and Lymph Nodes, Sua Yoo, et al, Int Jou Rad Onc, Bio, Phys, Volume 76, Issue 3, Pages 935-942, 1 March 2010).

This means a higher dose will be delivered to all neighboring critical structures such as the bladder, rectum, and sex organs (neurovascular bundles, penile bulb and proximal crus, which are the tissues that begin to form the penile shaft). With the arc system, the entire body receives a higher radiation dose, which may increase secondary malignancies and other complications in the long term.

The selling point with RapidArc™ for the manufacturer is that patients can be treated more quickly with the center employing a smaller support staff. But the crucial question is what the dose rate should be in order to safely eradicate cancer while sparing healthy tissue. We have serious reservations about this technology because changing the dose rate in this way may lead to deleterious outcomes over time.

To date, there are no clinical toxicity studies of RapidArc™. Such studies were not required for the manufacturer to win FDA approval. It may be that in the future arc therapy will be segmented and further developed to address these issues, although we believe that the rapid dose rate is dangerously high. At our institution, we have decided not to incorporate this technology in our DART systems arsenal because of our concerns about the extremely high dose rate. Even if the dose were segmented, it would still be extraordinarily high.

The arc technology will continue to be experimental for at least 5 to 10 years. As such, we are not convinced that RapidArc™ will be effective and not have detrimental late effects. Further long term studies are warranted and patients are advised to exercise caution with healthcare providers who promote RapidArc™. Doctors should be asked what long terms studies (10 years or more) they are relying on to vouch for the safety of this treatment modality.

A similarly untested delivery system, Elekta Infinity™ (and related products such as Elekta Unity and Elekta MR-Linac) is being marketed by a Swedish company, Elekta AB. Like RapidArc™, this form of Volumetric Modulated Arc Therapy must be considered experimental. The manufacturer describes its advantages as "speed and dose reduction," but the latter is still very much in question until long term data is available with regard to both efficacy and morbidity.

Since April 2010, Varian Medical Systems has been marketing another hi-tech system known as TrueBeam™ that is being combined with RapidArc™ at some centers, or combined with the Calypso 4D® Localization Tracking System (see discussion below) at other centers. Varian describes TrueBeam™ as a "platform for image-guided radiotherapy … the first fully-integrated system designed from the ground up to treat a moving target with unprecedented speed and accuracy." Those assertions really depend on how the TrueBeam™ system is integrated within the entire ensemble of IMRT treatment technology. When TrueBeam™ is combined with RapidArc™ or with Calypso 4D®, treatment time may be reduced to as little as 1-minute, but with the delivery of potentially dangerous high integral doses (that is, doses to normal surrounding tissue) required to accomplish that speed *it should be emphasized that none of these high dose rate systems, including TrueBeam™, have been sufficiently studied, so there is no long term clinical data.*

In fact, we use TrueBeam™ at our center, *without* Plus or RapidArc™, but in conjunction with many more 4D imaging techniques, including but not limited to, patient immobilization and motion tracking devices (including AlignRT and exact couch, 3rd Generation Cone Beam CT, Onboard Imaging, and Respiratory Gating). However, we do not speed up the treatment process by utilizing untested high dose rate protocols. It should be noted that combining the TrueBeam™ system with RapidArc™ or combining the Calypso 4D® system with TrueBeam™ or RapidArc™ does nothing to eliminate the uncertainties of these high dose rate systems. *Again, patients are advised to exercise caution until long-term studies from reputable* centers have been published in peer-reviewed journals to establish the safety and efficacy of Volumetric Modulated Arc Therapy.

This admonition includes the various combinations of these novel hi-tech systems being utilized in support of this experimental high dose rate approach. There are many acronyms but very few published studies. While most of these systems are FDA approved, it should be noted that the FDA approval mechanism for medical devices does not require the clinical trials that are mandatory for introducing new drugs to the marketplace. The lesson here once again is that until a therapeutic or technological innovation is proven in the long term with credible, peer reviewed data, "new" is not necessarily "better," despite the glowing sales hype of manufacturers and the often misleading advertizing campaigns of competing treatment centers.

What Is The Calypso® 4D Localization Tracking System?

The Calypso® 4D Localization System is an attempt to address the problem of organ motion in external radiation therapy by utilizing global positioning system (GPS) technology to track motion of the patient and prostate gland during daily radiation treatment sessions. According to the manufacturer, "Calypso Medical has developed a platform to objectively locate the tumor and monitoring tumor motion accurately and continuously without adding ionizing radiation." The Calypso® 4D Localization System consists of three components: the Calypso® 4D Localization System located in the treatment room; the Calypso® 4D Tracking Station located in the control room and Beacon® transponders, which are small wireless electromagnetic circuits designed for permanent implantation in the body.

The Seattle-based manufacturer, Calypso Medical Technologies, Inc, has been aggressively marketing the Calypso system and has recently developed strategic alliances with Varian Medical Systems, Siemens Healthcare, Elekta Corporation and Philips Medical. According to the manufacturer, the Beacon transponders interact with the Calypso System "to provide precise, continuous information on the location of the tumor during external beam radiation therapy. Any movement by the patient, including internal movement of the tumor, may cause the radiation to miss its intended target and hit adjacent healthy tissue. The real-time position information provided by the Calypso System allows physicians to deliver maximum radiation directly to the tumor while sparing the surrounding healthy tissues and organs from exposure" (from the Calypso Medical Web site–http://www.calypsomedical.com).

The concept sounds good, but the shortcoming not mentioned by the manufacturer is that the Calypso system is unable to alter the radiation beams in real time to take into consideration the movement it has tracked. In addition, Calypso doesn't actually track the "tumor," only the prostate, and the tumor may deform as the prostate moves. This system does not use respiratory gating, which tracks the motion of the prostate caused by breathing during treatment. With respiratory gating as part of our DART arsenal, we are able to hit the defined target each and every time the beam is activated. This level of assurance that the target is hit precisely, is only available with DART technology that is made possible by the complementary components of Respiratory Gating, Cone Beam Helical Tomography, 3D Cone Beam CT, On-board Imaging and the Exact Couch. Calypso employs none of these crucial modalities.

In comparing the Calypso® 4D System with the DART combined technique, it is important to note that our Varian 4D IG-IMRT technology is an integrated system that is a fully interfaced and delivers precise dosing of radiation to intraprostatic sites as well as the periprostatic margin and affected lymph nodes (as well as the bladder, rectum, neurovascular bundles, uro-genital diaphragm, penile bulb and proximate crus). DART as realized using all 4D IG-IMRT technologies accomplishes all of this in addition to accounting for organ motion in real time during the actual treatment, as well as real time dose optimization to intensify dose to specific targeted areas. It adjusts for dose to identified areas spontaneously while de-modulating (decreasing) the dose to surrounding critical structures.

Calypso, on the other hand, is essentially a piece of equipment that can be adapted to any existing linear accelerator. The Calypso system functions much like a gold seed marker in the prostate. The electromagnetic beacon transponders are placed into the prostate (2-3 of them) and they serve as a localization technique to track where the prostate is. It is then up to the radiation therapists (not the doctors) delivering the treatment to determine if the target is not being treated appropriately and the patient needs to be moved. This is not near the sophistication of an integrated system like DART, and can only account for prostate mobility. It cannot account for movement and identification of surrounding critical structures such as bladder and rectum, not to mention penile vessel anatomy, penile bulb, etc.

As part of the sales pitch for this guidance technique, the manufacturer promises "better treatment outcomes," but there is no long-term clinical data to support that claim. The most recent published study from Cedars-Sinai Medical Center on assessing side effects (morbidity) with the Calypso System (Sandler HM, et al. *Urology*, Volume 75, Issue 5, 1004-1008, May 2010), reports favorable results, but the follow-up time is only 2 months, which is hardly compelling data by the standards of cancer research. A recent study reported that the implantation of transponders during the procedure caused infectious complications in 10% of patients (Berglund RK, et al, BJU Int, 2012 Sep;110(6):834-9).

Our main concern with the Calypso system is with the risk of late side effects and secondary cancers, which require long-term clinical results for evaluation. As the Romans used to say, Caveat Emptor—Let the buyer beware.

What Is TomoTherapy®?

The TomoTherapy® Highly Integrated Adaptive Radiotherapy (HI-ART®) System is another form of radiation treatment delivered using CT guidance, both of which are continuous in nature and very slow, utilizing a rotational arc. The TomoTherapy system is manufactured by TomoTherapy Incorporated of Madison, Wisconsin. The system achieved FDA approval and first began treating patients in 2001, without having to undergo clinical trials to assess potential late toxicity or long term treatment outcomes.

With this system, the patient is often treated for 40 minutes, so the "BEAM-ON TIME" is enormous. This leads to "incident planned radiation," which then has a high integral dose because of the arc and the duration of treatment, with scattered photons and neutrons from the incident planned radiation, and the radiation from a continuously revolving CT Scan, which can also impart a sizeable dose to the entire body. As such, with this form of radiation treatment, we believe there is a high risk of developing secondary cancers. Indeed, TomoTherapy delivers such enormous doses of Total Body Radiation that it is not recommended in pediatric patients who have cancer (defined as patients in their twenties or less).

Once again, with this technology, there is no long term clinical data. Investigating late toxicity with Tomo-Therapy, a Canadian study reported that quality of life (QoL) within two years "with respect to bowel and sexual function was significantly affected" (Pervez N, et al, Curr Oncol, 2012 Jun;19(3):e201-10).

Those same researchers reported that at 5 years Grade 2 and Grade 3 late genitourinary toxicity was experienced in 17.0% and 2.44%, respectively (Pervez N, et al, Am J Clin Oncol. 2017 Apr;40(2):200-206).

Another short term Italian study reported late genitourinary toxicity at 6.6% and gastrointestinal toxicity at 5.3% of patients (Cuccia F, Hypofractionated postoperative helical tomotherapy in prostate cancer, Cancer Manag Res. 2018 Oct 29; 0:5053-5060).

In light of the high integral dose associated with arc therapy, we are not yet convinced that there is no significant risk of late side effects and secondary cancers with this system. Why would a 50-year-old patient or even a 60-year-old want to undergo TomoTherapy for prostate cancer only to risk being afflicted by leukemia or bladder cancer after 5 to 10 years?

In contrast, at our institution, we use "light speed" CT scans for diagnostics, which is accomplished in seconds. **ConeBeam CT** ("Tomography") involves real-time helical CT anatomical reconstruction of patient's anatomy to determine the actual daily delivered dose (also for Dynamic Adaptive Radiotherapy). This is an actual CT Cone Beam activated while the patient is being treated. Digital images are reconstructed by cone beam every 102 milliseconds (much like a camera with a rapid shutter speed, with an unbelievable mega-pixel resolution). We have a wireless real time system that enables physicians to watch what is happening with the patient in real time. We watch the treatment, and if we don't like what is happening, we halt the treatment with the touch of a button. So there is still the human touch to all of this advanced technology.

Our Cone Beam CT is also a "light speed" scanner so that the radiation dose is quantifiable, although small and safe. There may be some confusion because Cone Beam CT is often referred to as "Cone Beam CT Tomo Therapy," but it is really Cone Beam *Tomography*. It is not a form of treatment, but just one of our many image guidance tools used in conjunction with fully realized DART and all the technologies associated with 4D IG-IMRT.

What Are The Cyberknife® Robotic System and Hypofractionated Radiotherapy?

The Cyberknife® is essentially a linear accelerator mounted on a robotic arm. This modality was developed at Stanford in the 1990s, and the technology is manufactured by Accuray, Inc of Sunnyvale, California. While FDA-approved, the Cyberknife protocol is still considered investigational, with few published studies to date with more than 5 years of follow-up. At Stanford, Accuray's Cyberknife is now being combined with Varian Medical Systems' IG-IMRT technology. Cyberknife is also called "stereotactic body radiotherapy" (SBRT).

We have reservations about the Cyberknife based on its very penetrating radiation dose. The bottom line is that whenever you hypofractionate radiation (fewer treatments over a shorter time frame using higher radiation doses per treatment), you are making a compromise for the long haul. That is, expect significantly increased side effects over time. With prostate treatment, we're talking about progressive damage over time to the bladder, urethra, rectum, neurovascular bundles, etc. These symptoms will most likely begin to manifest in the long-term after treatment. The authors of a median 33-month follow-up Stanford study noted that longer term series would be needed to confirm "durable biochemical control rates and low late toxicity profiles" (Rad Onc, March 15, 2009,Volume 73, Issue 4, Pages 1043–1048).

"Why Would Anyone Choose Cyberknife?" This is the title of an entry on the Prostate Cancer Blog, posted in May 2007 by Dr. Louis Potters, founder of the New York Prostate Institute. Dr. Potters quotes an article in the International *Journal of Radiation Oncology, Biology and Physics* (vol. 67, No. 4, pp 1099) in which the author B.L. Madsen, M.D. writes that "in a Phase I/II trial of SHARP (Stereotactic Hypofractionated Accurate Radiotherapy for localize prostate cancer) the actuarial 48-month biochemical freedom from relapse is 70% using the ASTRO definition."

Dr. Potters should be aware that these results are not nearly as good as the results widely reported with DART and brachytherapy—with long-term data at the Dattoli Cancer Center (Dattoli MJ, et al, "Long-term outcomes for patients with prostate cancer having intermediate and high-risk disease, treated with combination external beam irradiation and brachytherapy," Journal of Oncology, July 2010).

A recent study by the Dana Farber Cancer Center, Brigham & Women's Hospital and Harvard Medical School cited two groundbreaking studies by Dr. Dattoli utilizing his treatment protocol that combines external radiation therapy (EBRT) with a brachytherapy boost. The Dana Farber study lamented the decline of brachytherapy in recent years because the data shows that seed implantation combined with external beam radiotherapy is by far the most effective treatment for prostate cancer (https://www.researchgate.net/publication/304104104_The_decreased_use_of_brachytherapyboostfor_intermediate_and_high-risk_prostate_cancer_despite_evidence_supporting_its_effectiveness).

A large multi-institutional study of 1100 patients treated with stereotactic body therapy reported that after 5-year follow-up, patients with low, intermediate and high-risk prostate cancer showed biochemical disease-free survival at 95%, 84% and 81%, respectively.

These are relatively short-term results, and the researchers did not use an absolute PSA nadir to determine success, thus inflating their data. The study did not report on side effects (King CR, et al, Radiother Oncol, 2013 Nov;109(2):217-21).

Similarly inconclusive results were reported with a more recent 8-year follow-up series, with low, intermediate and high-risk patients at 93.6, 84.3, and 65.0%. Again, this study did not report on toxicity (Katz A, et al, Fron Oncol, 2016 Jul 8;6:168). An earlier study by Georgetown University with 2-year follow-up reported serious genitourinary toxicity at 31% (Chen LN, et al, Radiat Oncol, 2013 Mar 13;8:58).

Without mincing words and pitting noted researchers against one another, the biggest obstacle facing Cyberknife (or Gammaknife or SHARP or any other such stereotactic hypofractionated therapy) for prostate cancer treatment is the lack of published, long-term clinical data to prove that it provides any better results than currently proven therapies. So why would anyone choose it? Convenience?

Facilities and physicians promoting Cyberknife have large investments to recoup. The marketing machines are grinding out stories and material to glorify their products. "Cyber" is a sexy word in advertising buzz today. And, while the therapy has been successfully used with treating intracranial tumors for years (typically for noncurative patients), its application for soft tissue tumors (such as prostate) is glorified as "new"—as if everything "new" is "better."

Website material from the manufacturer of the Cyberknife touts its ability to achieve clinical flexibility, delineation of tumor versus normal tissue for targeting, shorter treatment time and relatively low toxicity of the rectum and bladder. But beware. One physician at a large Cyberknife facility in Oklahoma in an Internet patient support forum admits that "generally speaking, failure (at least in our hands) occurs most often when all our imaging does not make it possible to determine where the tumor stops and the normal tissue starts. We usually err on the side of including more volume, but sometimes we just can't make the correct decision. We have sometimes been able to go back and re-treat the area we missed." The link for this reference is http://www.cyberknifesupport.org/forum/default.aspx?f=16&m=5736.

A primary goal of combination therapy (DART and seeds) at the Dattoli Cancer Center is to stop the identified tumor in its tracks, but the larger ultimate goal is to treat the entire gland. We know that whatever biochemical forces were in place to cause the growth of the primary tumor are at work, albeit at a slower pace, throughout the gland. All the intense focal efforts to treat only the tumor are leaving the rest of the gland untouched—and ripe for future cancer growth.

With DART enabled by 4D IG-IMRT and subsequent Palladium-103 brachytherapy, we are able to sculpt the radiation dose to surround the gland and spare the central core housing the urethra—attacking the active tumor cells and rendering the remainder of gland fallow for future tumor growth. It is our goal to have prostate cancer be a one-time event in the man's life.

Cyberknife proponents herald their 5-day treatment vs the 28-day DART program, as "more convenient" for the patient. How "convenient," we ask, will it be for the patient to face a repeat performance 3, 4, 8 or more years down the road? Or how convenient will it be in the long run (late effects of radiation) when patients develop urethral and/or rectal fistulas, bladder damage, rectal ulcerations or perforations requiring colostomies, hip and bone necrosis—which are all well documented complications from hypofractionated radiation in its various forms?

Hyprofractionated forms of radiotherapy such as Cyberknife, HDR, and Hypofractionated IMRT are characterized as either moderate and extreme (or ultra) depending on the dose and number of treatments. The published guidelines of the American Society of Clinical Oncology recommend that physicians should counsel patients about the limited follow-up beyond five years for most studies evaluating hypofractionation and the increased risk of acute and late toxicity with Moderately Hypofractionated IMRT compared to Conventional IMRT.

The guidelines suggest Ultra-Hypofractionated Radiotherapy should be limited to clinical trials due to the risk of late toxicity (Morgan SC, Hypofractionated Radiation Therapy for Localized Prostate Cancer: Executive Summary of an ASTRO, ASCO, and AUA Evidence-Based Guideline, Pract Radiatt Oncol, 2018 Nov–Dec;8(6):354-360).

Proton Beam Therapy (PBT) vs DART With Brachytherapy: Which Is Best For Treating Prostate Cancer?

Radiation therapy in all its forms utilizes atomic or subatomic particles: electrons, protons, neutrons and photons, which include x-rays and gamma rays. These particles differ in terms of charge, mass and other physical characteristics. Like visible light, the energy of conventional x-ray radiation takes the form of photons. Radiation therapies utilizing proton and neutron beams have been developed in

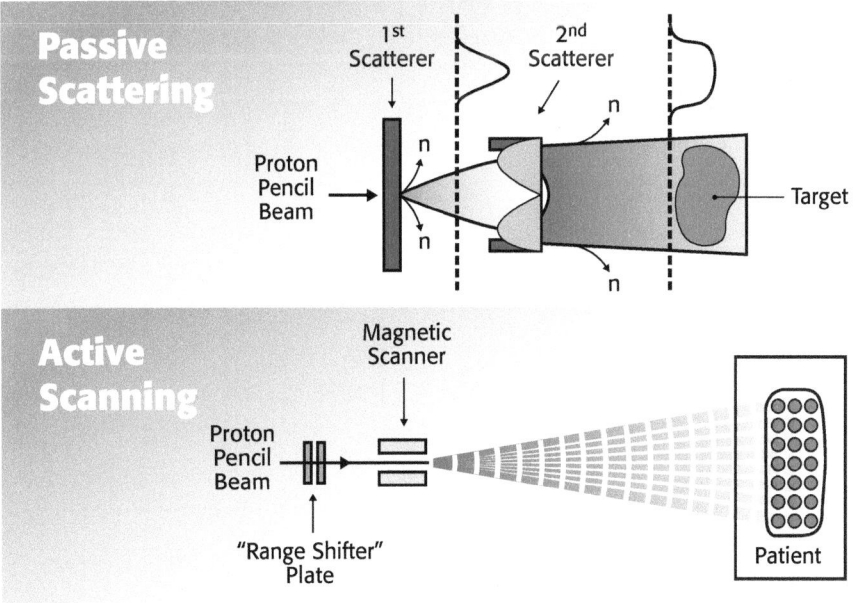

the hope that they might offer some advantage over conventional photon beams. Heavy carbon ions are even more massive than protons and neutrons and are also being investigated as particle beam therapy for prostate cancer.

Protons and neutrons are generated by proton accelerators rather than the linear accelerators that are used to generate photons. Each type of radiation therapy delivers a dose of highly energized particles that interact in various ways with the tissue they traverse. In the case of x-rays and protons, a process called ionization causes electrons to be displaced in the atoms of DNA molecules in cancer cells. This interaction damages the DNA and causes cell death. The strategy of targeting tumors with cancer-killing doses of radiation is essentially the same regardless of which kind of radiation is used.

Unlike other forms of radiation like x-rays that begin releasing their energy as soon as they enter the body, protons travel through bodily tissues initially releasing very little energy, but at a certain calculable point, the energy that the beam delivers rises dramatically to a peak, known as the Bragg peak. The Bragg peak is like the focus of a magnifying lens, and allows the radiation to be targeted to the site of the tumor. Protons may appear at first to have some theoretical advantage over photons because they can be accurately focused to release most of their ionizing energy at a certain depth to encompass a calculated tumor volume, while avoiding nearby healthy organs. By contrast, the depth at which photons deposit their maximal energy is determined by the energy levels of the photons and can range from the skin surface to a depth of approximately 6 centimeters.

The use of Proton Therapy for the treatment of prostate cancer in particular has become increasingly controversial because of questions about its efficacy and the multimillion dollar expense of constructing proton beam cyclotrons.

The June 2008 issue of Oncology Journal (Volume 33, Number 7, pp. 748-753) offered an assessment of the heated battle between protons and photons. The article was authored by radiation oncologists at Harvard Medical School, the first institution in the world to utilize proton therapy (primarily for small brain tumors). The authors suggested at the time, "There is a growing interest in the use of proton therapy for the treatment of many cancers. While much evidence supports this notion in context of many oncologic sites, only limited clinical data have compared protons to photons in prostate cancer. Therefore, the increasing enthusiasm for the use of protons in prostate cancer has aroused considerable concern. Some have questioned its ability to limit morbidity. Theoretical concerns over potential additional risks for developing secondary malignancies (ie, cancer in other areas of the body), as well as promoting hip fractures."

While the use of proton beam therapy (PBT) to treat prostate cancer patients more than doubled from 2004 to 2012, the controversies surrounding protons and prostate cancer has continued to the present without resolution. In 2016 researchers at Harvard Medical School published another study on the use of proton therapy for prostate cancer that concluded, "Long-term follow-up is needed to determine whether the increased use of proton therapy for prostate cancer is justified."

The Size of the Proton Beam Requires "Scattering" to treat Prostate Cancer

We believe that the best use for protons is in the treatment of tiny brain tumors, and not for treating a gland the size of the prostate. Because protons travel in tiny, straight beams they must be "scattered" to form a large enough beam to treat the entire area of the prostate. In passive scattering, or "passive modulation" (the most common proton method utilized), "scattering foils" are added to produce a beam of large enough size to cover the entire target. Unfortunately, once the proton beam encounters the filter or scanner, it becomes cone-shaped and results in spreading the radiation dose outside of and beyond the target area. In other words, the beam cannot be manipulated into a spherical shape as can be done with the photon beam (or IMRT) using "multi-leaf collimators," which allow the microbeams to be precisely sculpted. In fact, none of that sophisticated technology (e.g. 4D IGRT) is used for protons and many patients are being treated with older 3D Conformal Radiation with protons used as a boost, combining photons and protons.

Eric J. Hall, D.Phil, D.Sc, of Columbia University, widely regarded as the world's premiere radiobiologist, writing in *The International Journal of Radiation Oncology, Biology and Physics* (2006;65:1-7), described the thorny technical challenge of harnessing proton beams to treat prostate cancer that has characterized the past ten years: "Protons emerging from a cyclotron form a narrow pencil beam. To cover a treatment field of practical size, the beam must be either scattered by a foil or scanned. Passive scanning is by far the simplest technique but suffers the disadvantage of increased total-body effective dose to the patient... Passive modulation results in effective doses distant from the field edge that are 10 times higher than those characteristic of IMRT."

Dr. Hall also suggested that "the scattering foil becomes a source of neutrons, which results in a total-body dose to the patient." Because of this widening cone-shaped beam, the potential side effects with protons will be greater even at lower dose levels than with our high energy photons, which is opposite of what many patients currently are being told by proponents of proton therapy.

Protons Versus Photons: Which Is State Of The Art?

Many people believe that proton therapy causes significantly fewer complications than does traditional external radiation therapy (EBRT), which utilizes photons. However, the newest technology in external radiation therapy with photons surpasses both proton therapy and traditional external radiation therapy. The DART treatment protocol enabled by all methods of 4D IG-IMRT allows for "inverse treatment planning" utilized for the initial IMRT planning phase.

With DART, inverse treatment planning provides the radiation oncologist with the ability to plan for and control the amount of radiation received by the tissues surrounding the prostate while maximizing the dose to the prostate. Thereafter, a number of technological advances, including but not limited to Cone Beam Tomography, Exact Couch ™, Portal Vision, On-Board Imaging, AlignRT, CT SIM+™ with RapidSIM™, and Respiratory Gating are combined to allow for the analysis of organ motion in real-time (the 4th dimension) to achieve unsurpassed accuracy. Once the motion is detected, numerous software programs activate to adapt the radiation to target the organ site which may have moved.

This is true Dynamic Adaptive Radiotherapy (DART). Using gating technologies, DART can even hit a continually moving target! This ability to optimize and adapt to changes is the basis for DART. As explained below, none of this is even remotely possible with protons.

It should be emphasized that the radio-biological effects (RBE) or cancer killing ability of photons in the high dose range used at our institute with DART are identical to that of protons. This being the case, we strongly favor DART because of the highly sophisticated beam arrangements which are available here, state-of-the-art prostate targeting, as outlined above, and far more mature research data which has been accrued with high energy photons in general compared to the relatively short history of protons.

Dr. Anthony Zeitman of the Harvard Medical School summed up the situation with protons for *Oncology Times* ("Proton Beam Radiation Therapy: Balancing Evidence-Based Use with the Bottom Line," April 25, 2010). As of this writing, his words still hold true in light of all the studies we have seen to date: "I believe during this last decade that technology has proceeded at an incredible pace, but that doesn't necessarily mean better patient care. We exist in a very competitive medical environment, and over the last 10 years technology has been a way hospitals brand themselves, the way they sell themselves with billboards on the highway announcing they have proton beam therapy or perhaps a Cyberknife. We should be masters of technology, but technology has become our master and an end in itself, and many of these technologies are being widely used I expect because they are prestige projects for marketing purposes without proof of real benefit. They may be beneficial, but no one has proven it in some cases, and this is really a very deeply disturbing aspect of contemporary medicine."

A British study entitled "Current clinical evidence for proton therapy," reported... a systematic review of published peer-reviewed literature [on proton therapy] reported previously and updated here is devoid of any clinical data demonstrating benefit in terms of survival, tumor control, or toxicity in comparison with best conventional treatment for any of the tumors so far treated..." (Brada et al, (Cancer J. 2009 Jul-Aug;15(4):319-24).

Published research studies have already demonstrated advantages of IMRT over 3-D conformal radiation at higher dose levels. Meanwhile, a number of studies have even demonstrated the lack of superiority of protons over 3D conformal radiation. We are unaware of any proton study series utilizing significantly higher doses than 3D conformal radiation. It should also be noted that with most proton studies to date, protons are combined with external radiation (photons) in order to increase the dose. This approach is known as a "proton boost."

The preponderance of data suggests that higher doses equal higher cure rates. It is not yet possible to safely escalate protons to doses as high as those used with DART coupled with a Palladium-103 brachytherapy. It has been well documented that it requires far higher doses of radiation to truly eradicate prostate cancer. At this point, this degree of dose escalation has been accomplished only with DART and Pd-103 brachytherapy, which also has the advantage of maximally sparing adjacent normal tissues. Neither of those goals has been achieved with protons.

How effective Is The High Energy Photon Beam Used In DART / 4D IG-IMRT Compared to The Proton Beam?

With the effective radiation dose around the prostate using DART, we are able to control and modulate the beam in such a way that 'structures within structures' can receive a lower or higher dose while maintaining an adequate dose to the target area (the prostate plus a margin, or possibly even lymph nodes). For example, the urethra receives far lower dose than the surrounding prostate tissue, while the tumor areas receive a much higher dose than the surrounding prostate tissue.

With proton beam therapy, as mentioned, there is always a need for a "compensating filter" in order to expand the beam width to treat the prostate to appropriate dose levels. In doing so, control over the modulation of the beam is compromised to the extent that it becomes impossible to accurately target small areas within the prostate to receive lower or higher doses, as is possible with 4D IG-IMRT (through the complementary treatment planning processes known as "dose escalation" and "dose demodulating").

Therefore, with protons, the entire prostate receives essentially the same dose and this dose is significantly less than what can be achieved with 4D IG-IMRT. While the overall dose to the prostate with DART / 4D IG-IMRT may look similar to proton therapy, the ability to control the dose to the critical structures within the target (prostate) is lost with protons. These functional results from proton filtering or scanning make 4D IG-IMRT a more versatile and therefore superior treatment compared to proton therapy.

Additionally, because of the need for the "compensating filter," the normal adjacent tissues including the bladder and rectum through which the proton beam enters the pelvis receive far higher dose than with 4D IG-IMRT. Again, this is quite the opposite of what many patients are being told by proton therapy practitioners.

What the Research on Protons Tells Us

Researchers at Loma Linda University published the first large series on outcomes with proton therapy for 1255 prostate cancer patients (524 received PBT alone and 731 were treated with conformal radiation with a proton boost). The study included patients with low, intermediate and high-risk cancer. After 8 years of patient follow-up, biochemical disease-free survival was 73% overall, hardly impressive compared to contemporary published results for IMRT and brachytherapy (Slater JD, et al, *Int J Radiat Oncol Biol Phys*. 2004 Jun 1;59(2):348-52).

A study by Massachusetts General Hospital reported on early stage prostate cancer patients treated with high dose (79.2 Gy) proton beam therapy. With 10-year follow-up, biochemical disease free survival was only 83.3%, significantly lower than published results achieved from our center and other leading IMRT groups (Zeitman AL et al, J Clin Oncol, 2010 Mar 1;28(7):1106-11).

Researchers at the same institution have also demonstrated that patients undergoing high-dose proton therapy (82 Gy) at 18 months experience a rate of 7% severe genitourinary-gastrointestinal side effects, RTOG Grade 3, late toxicity (Coen JJ, et al, Int Radiat Oncol Biol Phys, 2011 Nov 15;81(4):1005-9.

By contrast, Memorial Sloan Kettering researchers reported the likelihood of Grade 3 toxicity was 3% for men undergoing high dose IMRT (81 Gy) with 8-year follow-up (Zelefsky MJ, et al, J Urol, 2006 Oct;176(4 Pt 1):1415-9). In our own published DART-brachytherapy series, there were no cases of Grade 3 or Grade 4 toxicity.

With proton therapy, rectal bleeding is also a common toxicity, and the risk correlates with the volume of the rectum receiving 70 to 75 Gy. Proton therapy is not expected to lower risk of rectal bleeding because it does not reduce the volume of the rectum receiving high doses of radiation compared with IMRT.

A study by the University of Florida Proton Therapy Institute reported that as many as 32.3% of patients experienced rectal toxicity (Grades 1-3) after PBT (Colaco RJ et al, Int J Radiat Onco Biol Phys, 2015 Jan 1;91(1):172-81).

Similarly, urinary toxicities like urethritis, urethral strictures and cystitis generally occur with PBT because of exposure of the urethra and/or bladder neck to higher doses of radiation than with Image-Guided IMRT. A 2013 retrospective Medicare database study by the Yale University School of Medicine reported that one year after treatment with proton beam therapy, 18.8% of patients experienced genitourinary side effects.

That same study also reported on the disparity of costs for therapy, with proton beam therapy receiving $32,428 in Medicare reimbursement versus $18,575 for IMRT (Yu JB, J Natl Cancer Inst, 2013 Jan 2;105(1):25-32).

Researchers at the University of North Carolina showed that overall genitourinary toxicity with protons was significantly higher than with IMRT (approximately 17% for PBT and 12% for IMRT (Sheets, NC, et al, JAMA, 2012 Apr 18;307(15):1611-20).

Several clinical trials are now underway comparing proton beam therapy with IMRT, including a Phase III randomized trial of proton beam therapy vs. IMRT for low and intermediate-risk prostate cancer (clinicaltrials.gov ID NCT01617161). Long-term results from that trial are not expected for some years.

Given our current knowledge and in light of the various risk factors, patients are advised to exercise caution when considering proton therapy and other high-dose radiotherapies without evidence based-data and long-term published clinical results.

As this booklet goes to press, there is news that some major insurance carriers are denying reimbursement for Proton Beam Therapy for prostate cancer, based on its lack of demonstrable benefit over photon therapies (equivalent survival), increased gastrointestinal morbidity compared to photon radiation, and its enormous cost differential.

What Is Neutron Beam Therapy And How Does It Compare With Other Forms of Radiation?

The basic effect of ionizing radiation is to disrupt the ability of cells to divide and grow by damaging their DNA strands. With photons and protons, the damage is done primarily by activated radical ions produced by atomic interactions involving electrons orbiting the nucleus of the atom. Because of the nature of these characteristic interactions, photon and proton radiation are referred to as low linear energy transfer (low LET) radiation. With neutron therapy, also called Fast Neutron Radiation Therapy (FNRT), the damage to the DNA is done primarily by nuclear interactions. Neutrons are referred to as high linear energy transfer (high LET) radiation. Tumor cells damaged by high LET radiation (neutrons) are less able to repair themselves and continue to grow than are tumor cells damaged by low LET radiation (photons and protons).

In addition, unlike low LET photons and protons, neutrons do not depend on oxygen to damage the DNA in cancer cells and cause cell death. Therefore, neutron beam therapy may have a certain theoretical advantage over conventional photon radiation because high LET neutrons might be more effective against large, bulky tumors that typically have low oxygen levels (hypoxic) near the center of their mass. This characteristic of neutrons might afford some benefit when treating these larger tumors that are more resistant to low LET radiation and to hormonal therapy. But that theoretical possibility has never been demonstrated clinically.

The radiobiological effect of neutrons is so high that the required prescription dose is about one-third the dose required with photons or protons. As such, a full course of neutron therapy is carried out with only 10 to 12 treatments, compared to 30 to 40 treatments needed for conventional photon radiation. Neutrons are sometimes combined with a reduced course of standard photon radiation therapy. Clinical trials of neutrons have suggested that they may be more effective against advanced prostate cancers than is conventional radiation; however, these results are still considered short-term. It should also be noted that because neutrons are such a highly penetrating form of radiation, they have also been shown to result in a far greater risk of complications than conventional radiation therapy.

Patients considering neutron therapy should be aware that it is still investigational without any compelling long-term clinical data to support its use versus the most advanced photon radiation therapy (DART and 4D IG-IMRT). Here again with neutrons, we are concerned with the risk of late side effects and secondary cancers. The following studies assess the efforts of researchers attempting to adapt neutrons to the treatment of prostate cancer, faced with the challenge of reducing the neutron radiation dose to normal tissue:

Snyder M, et al, "Dose escalation in prostate cancer using intensity modulated neutron radiotherapy," Radiother Oncol, 2011 May;99(2):201-6.

Santanam L, "Intensity modulated neutron radiotherapy for the treatment of adenocarcinoma of the prostate," Int J Radiat Oncol Biol Phys. Aug, 2007.

Forman JD, et al., "Fast neutron irradiation for prostate cancer," Cancer Metastasis Rev. 2002;21(2):131-5.

What Are The Treatment Options if External Radiation Fails?

Patients who are not cured by any of the various forms of external radiation therapy have several options for salvage therapy, including radical surgery. As mentioned, the operation to remove the prostate is more difficult after radiation. Many doctors do not recommend salvage prostatectomy because of their own limited experience. They will inform the patient that the risk of complications is high, while the likelihood of cure is relatively low. Nonetheless, this remains a viable option in experienced surgical hands.

A second treatment with radiation is usually not advised since the first course of radiation did not cure the cancer and the risk of complications is high. There has been, however, a growing interest in treating failed external radiation patients with brachytherapy, since seed implant radiation can be focused on the prostate, with less risk of damage to the rectum and surrounding tissue. One recent study reported that as many as 50% of these salvage brachytherapy patients were disease-free at 5 years. Patients who have had combination therapy with both external radiation and brachytherapy would not be advised to have any additional radiation (see "What are the Treatment Options if Combined Radiotherapy Fails?")

Cryosurgery is a primary treatment method that involves the insertion of freezing probes into the prostate to kill cancerous tissue. This technique has also been used as a salvage therapy for locally recurrent prostate cancer after failed radiation, though there is little published data available. One study reported a disease-free survival rate of 74% after two years, but with a very high rate of complications such as incontinence and erectile dysfunction. This incontinence rate is dramatically reduced in experienced hands.

Over the past decade, a more limited application of cryosurgery known as "focal prostate cryoblation has been investigated as both a primary and salvage therapy. This technique involves partial ablation of the gland with freezing and is aimed at treating the primary tumor while sparing healthy tissue in the gland and surrounding structures. Some cryosurgeons refer to this technique as "prostate lumpectomy." Patients eligible for this approach are usually limited to those having unilateral prostate cancer (tumor confined to one lobe).

A recent study from the Cleveland Clinic demonstrated modestly favorable results when salvage focal cryosurgery was utilized to treat patients with recurrent cancer after various forms of radiotherapy. With patient follow-up of 1, 3, and 5 years, researchers reported biochemical disease-free survival rates of 95.3%, 72.4%, and 46.5%. Erectile function was retained by 50% of patients, while 5.5% experienced urinary incontinence requiring them to wear absorbent pads. Another 6.6% of men suffered from urinary retention after therapy (Li YH, Prostate, 2015 Jan;75(1):1-7).

If a man's PSA after external radiation (or brachytherapy) rises only very slowly over a period of one to three years, then the cancer may still be confined within the prostate. These patients have the most options of patients who fail with radiation, including active surveillance (AS). A number of studies have shown that there are patients with biopsy-detected local recurrence who have survived 10 years or more without experiencing any progression of the disease. However, more aggressive tumors with Gleason scores of 7 to 10 may secrete little PSA, and even a slow PSA rise may be significant with respect to tumor growth and cancer spread.

In addition to salvage treatments like brachytherapy, surgery and cryosurgery, there is also the option of hormonal therapy. The same considerations that apply to hormonal therapy after failed surgery apply to hormonal therapy for men with local or distant cancer recurrence after radiation. Some studies suggest that men treated with a combination of hormones and radiation as their initial treatment have a reduced rate of failure. However, initial radical prostatectomy coupled with hormones have not demonstrated a similar benefit.

With the object of shutting down the body's production of testosterone completely, many doctors combine drugs like Lupron® (or Eligard® or Zoladex® or TRELSTAR®) with Casodex®, which together provide a total blockage against the male hormones that nourish prostate cancer. For many men, the use of this type of combination hormonal therapy to achieve a castration level of testosterone that may slow the progression of the disease is certainly preferable to undergoing surgical castration (orchiectomy), which is a less expensive way to achieve the same end. In addition, unlike surgical castration, this form of medical castration is reversible and may be used intermittently. The patients may be on hormones 6 to 12 months, and then completely off hormones until the PSA reaches a predetermined value. This allows for recovery of the male bodily functions.

What are The Treatment Options if Brachytherapy Fails?

Patients who have had seed implantation without initial success have the option of being re-seeded. Although long term results are not yet available, this approach appears to be promising, and typically involves using a different isotope the second time around. If the patient was first implanted with iodine, then palladium might be used as a salvage therapy in the hope that the cancer will be more sensitive to the second isotope. If the first implant was technically mishandled, then a second implant affords the opportunity of correcting misplacements that may have caused underdosing. In some cases, high dose rate (HDR) temporary implants may be used if permanent implants fail.

Patients who have undergone combination therapy with both external radiation and brachytherapy would not be advised to have additional radiation as a salvage therapy because the initial combined course of radiation did not cure the cancer and there would be a high risk of side effects.

Patients who underwent brachytherapy as a monotherapy and who experience treatment failure also have the salvage options of surgery, cryosurgery, hormonal therapy, and watchful waiting. In some cases, several months of hormonal therapy may be prescribed to reduce the size of the tumor prior to an attempt at salvage therapy with either surgery or cryosurgery (focal cryosurgery if the recurrence is limited to one lobe). Patients may also consider bio-thermia, which combines cryosurgery and hyperthermia. High Intensity Frequency Ultrasound is another option, and as noted, researchers are working on a number of immunotherapy vaccines for which there are clinical trials underway.

What are the Treatment Options if Combined Radiotherapy Fails?

Patients who have undergone combination therapy utilizing both external radiation and brachytherapy would not be advised to have any form of additional radiation, because the initial combined radiation protocol did not cure the cancer and there would be a high risk of side effects.

Patients who experience recurrence after combined radiotherapy have salvage options that may include surgery, crysosurgery, hormonal therapy, biothermia, High Intensity Frequency Ultrasound (HIFU) and possibly Active Surveillance (AS).

APPENDIX A

Dr. Dattoli
On the Case for
Brachytherapy

For men with intermediate and high-risk prostate cancer, some of the strongest evidence in modern radiation oncology supports the combination of external beam radiation therapy (EBRT) and brachytherapy (radioactive seed implantation). The landmark ASCEND-RT trial, first published in 2017 and updated in 2023, demonstrated a 50% reduction in recurrence when a low-dose-rate brachytherapy boost was added to dose-escalated EBRT.

At 10 years, Ascende-RT reported approximately 85% of patients receiving the brachytherapy boost remained free from biochemical progression — a dramatic and clinically meaningful improvement over EBRT alone.

In oncology, it is rare to see an intervention cut recurrence risk in half. Yet despite this level of randomized evidence, brachytherapy is recommended less frequently today than it was a decade ago.

The Real Issue: A Training Gap

The reason that brachytherapy is not widely recommended is not a lack of data but a lack of training. Over the past 15 to 20 years, many radiation oncology residency and fellowship programs have significantly reduced hands-on training in prostate brachytherapy. As fewer trainees graduate with procedural experience, fewer practitioners feel comfortable offering the technique.

When physicians are not trained in a procedure, it is less likely to be recommended — even when the evidence strongly supports it. This has created a widening gap between what the data demonstrate and what many patients are told by their doctors. Brachytherapy is not an outdated therapy. It is under-taught and under-trained.

Long-Term Data Defining True Success

Randomized, controlled data are powerful. But long-term follow-up is what ultimately defines durability. Our own published outcomes have appeared in peer-reviewed journals including *Cancer, Journal of Oncology, Brachytherapy*, and the *International Journal of Radiation Oncology Biology Physics* (known as the Red Journal). Our published data extend well beyond 16 years of follow-up and represent some of the longest combined-modality prostate cancer data reported in the modern era.

Our findings demonstrate the following:

- Near 100% local control
- Durable biochemical disease-free survival
- Sustained cancer control across intermediate- and high-risk groups
- Outcomes measured in decades, not just years

Prostate cancer has a long natural history. Five-year results are reassuring. Ten-year results are meaningful. Outcomes extending beyond 16 years begin to define true oncologic durability. When local control is maximized, recurrence declines. When recurrence declines, the risk of metastatic progression falls. When durable control is achieved, salvage therapy can be avoided. Indeed, long-term data can change the trajectory of disease.

Why the Combination Works

The biological rationale for the combination radiation treatment modality is straightforward. External beam radiation treats the prostate and the surrounding at-risk tissues, especially lymph nodes. At our center, this is delivered as Dynamic Adaptive Radiotherapy (DART), allowing precision targeting and adaptive dose optimization. Brachytherapy then delivers an intensified, highly conformal radiation dose directly inside the prostate – where the cancer resides.

This combined approach achieves:

- Higher intraprostatic dose escalation
- Steeper dose gradients
- Superior tumoricidal intensity
- Relative sparing of surrounding structures

Dose matters in the treatment of prostate cancer. But how the dose is delivered matters even more. Dose-escalated EBRT alone simply cannot replicate the intra-prostatic dose distribution achieved with brachytherapy.

Experience Is a Determinant of Outcome

Brachytherapy is technically demanding. It requires precision, judgment, and procedural repetition. I have performed more prostate brachytherapy procedures than any physician in the world. That experience translates into consistency of technique, optimized dosimetry, and reproducible long-term outcomes.

At the Dattoli Cancer Center, we integrate DART external beam radiation and brachytherapy under one roof, within our own surgical suite. This model ensures:

- Seamless coordination of care
- Unified treatment planning
- Technical consistency
- Direct physician accountability

Patients are not referred elsewhere for part of their treatment. The entire strategy and treatment plan are designed and delivered cohesively.

Medicine evolves. Technologies change. Training patterns shift. But evidence remains the foundation of responsible care. When a well-run randomized trial like ASCEND-RT demonstrates a 50% reduction in recurrence, that finding demands attention. When long-term follow-up extending beyond 16 years confirms durable control and near-100% local control, that evidence-based data demands both attention and respect.

The decline in brachytherapy utilization does not reflect inferior outcomes. It reflects a generational shift in training exposure. Patients deserve to know the difference. Physicians have an obligation to recommend therapies supported by the strongest available data — even when those therapies require technical specialization.

The case for brachytherapy is not nostalgic.

- It is statistical.
- It is biological.
- It is longitudinal.
- It is durable.

And when performed with expertise, it remains one of the most powerful tools in prostate cancer treatment.

To Our Patients — Present and Future

If you are facing a prostate cancer diagnosis, you deserve complete information. You deserve to know which treatments have demonstrated control measured not just in years, but in decades.

You deserve to know when a therapy has been shown to cut recurrence risk in half. And you deserve to receive care in a center where both advanced external beam radiation and brachytherapy are delivered seamlessly, cohesively, and with unmatched procedural experience.

At the Dattoli Cancer Center, we offer brachytherapy not because it is traditional, but because the evidence supports it, our outcomes validate it, and long-term cancer control is the standard our patients expect. Prostate cancer treatment should not be limited by training trends. It should be guided by data, experience, and a relentless commitment to durable, long-term cure.

That is the case for brachytherapy boost combined with DART.

References

1 Justin Oh, et al., An Updated Analysis of the Survival Endpoints of ASCENDE-RT, *Int J Radiat Oncol Biol Phys*, 2023 Apr 1;115(5):1061-1070.

2 Rodda S, Tyldesley S, Morris WJ, et al. ASCENDE-RT: Treatment-related morbidity analysis comparing LDR brachytherapy boost to EBRT boost. *Int J Radiat Oncol Biol Phys*.2017;98(2):286-295.

3 Morris WJ, Tyldesley S, Rodda S, et al. ASCENDE-RT: Analysis of survival endpoints for a randomized trial comparing a low-dose-rate brachytherapy boost with dose-escalated external beam boost for high- and intermediate-risk prostate cancer. *Int J Radiat Oncol Biol Phys*. 2017;98(2):275-285.

4 Dattoli M, Wallner K, True L, Cash J, Sorace R. Long-term outcomes after treatment with brachytherapy and supplemental conformal radiation for prostate cancer patients having intermediate and high-risk features. *Cancer*. 2007;110(3):551-555.

5 Dattoli M, Wallner K, True L, Bostwick D, Cash J, Sorace R. Long-term outcomes for patients with prostate cancer treated with combination external beam irradiation and brachytherapy. *J Oncol*.2010;2010:471375.

First Published *Journey Express*, Spring 2026

APPENDIX B

STATE OF THE ART BRACHYTHERAPY, IMRT AND DART

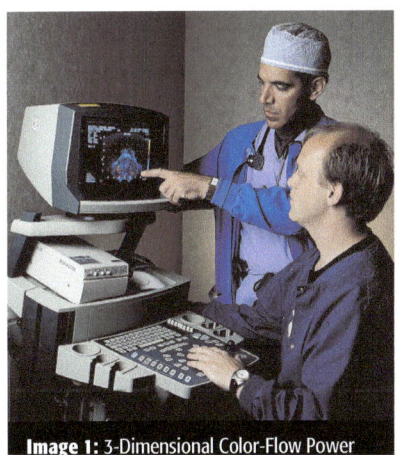

Image 1: 3-Dimensional Color-Flow Power Doppler Ultrasound used to image cancer areas inside and outside the prostate gland.

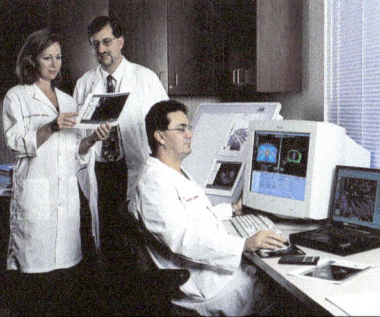

Image 2: The computer center for planning and customizing the best treatment programs utilizing brachytherapy and 4-Dimensional Image Guided-Intensity Modulated Radiation Therapy (4D IG-IMRT).

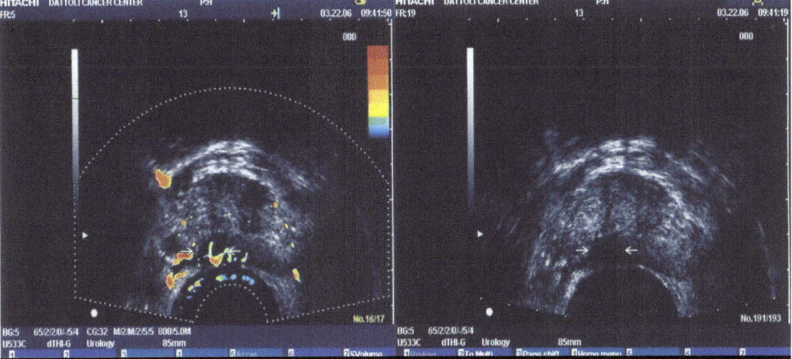

Image 3: Comparison of Color-Flow Power Doppler Ultrasound image (left) with conventional gray-scale ultrasound image (right) of the same patient. Note: The bright red areas in the Color-Flow Power Doppler image reveal the location of suspected cancer sites, which are not visible using gray-scale ultrasound imaging.

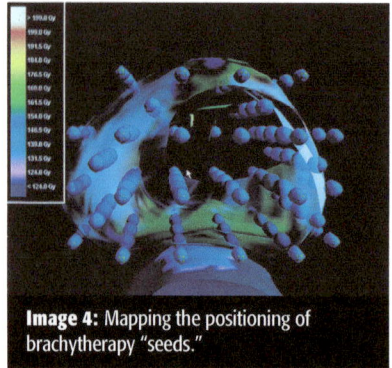

Image 4: Mapping the positioning of brachytherapy "seeds."

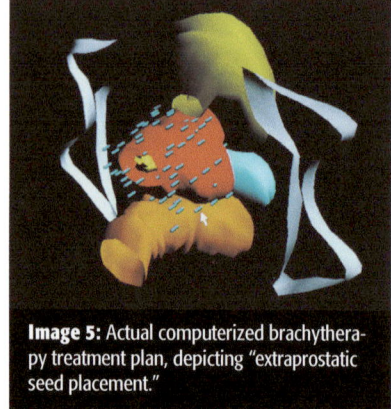

Image 5: Actual computerized brachytherapy treatment plan, depicting "extraprostatic seed placement."

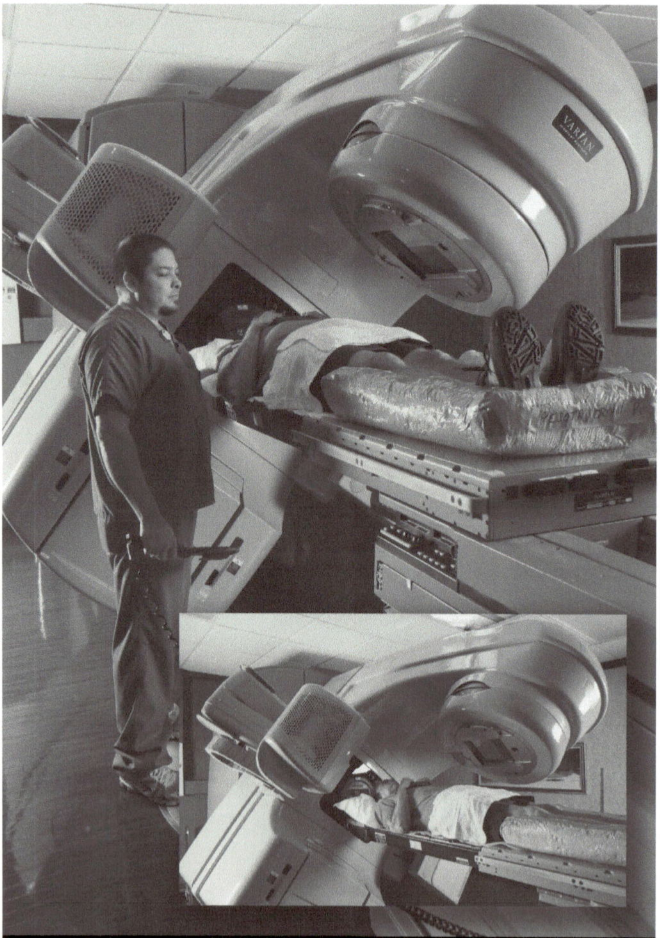

Image 6: DART in action. A patient being treated with the Varian 4D IG-IMRT Linear Accelerator

APPENDIX B: STATE OF THE ART BRACHYTHERAPY, IMRT AND DART

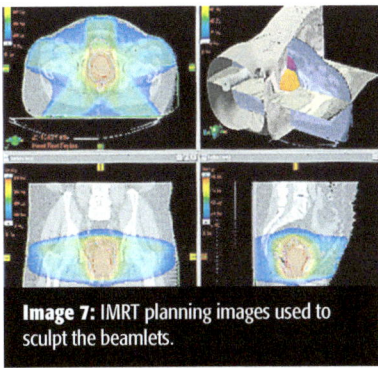

Image 7: IMRT planning images used to sculpt the beamlets.

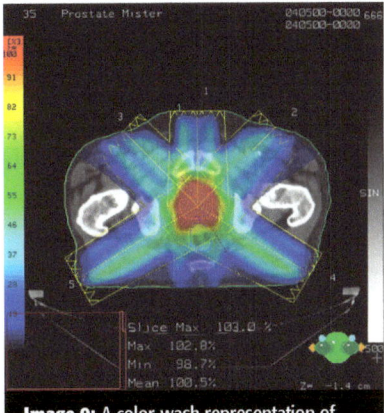

Image 8: An IMRT plan for treating prostate cancer, concentrating the radiation dose in the tumor (red) while avoiding the nearby bladder (yellow) and rectum (green). Courtesy of Varian Medical Systems.

Image 9: A color-wash representation of an IMRT plan, showing how the radiation dose will be distributed in and around the prostate. The area of high dose (red) corresponds tightly to the tumor area being treated. Courtesy of Varian Medical Systems.

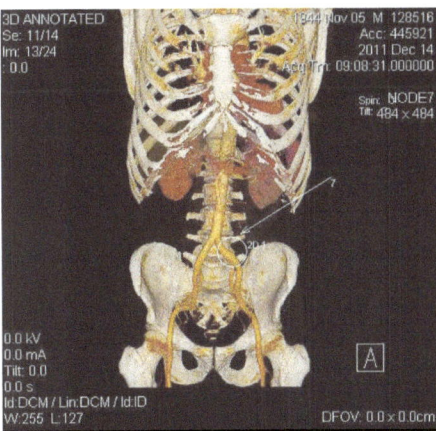
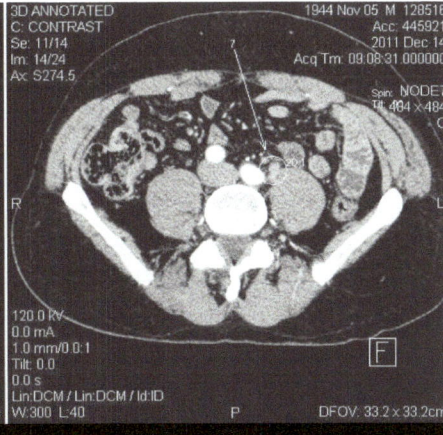

Image 10: A Dynamic Contrast Enhanced MRI study for the identification of cancer metastasis in the lymph nodes.

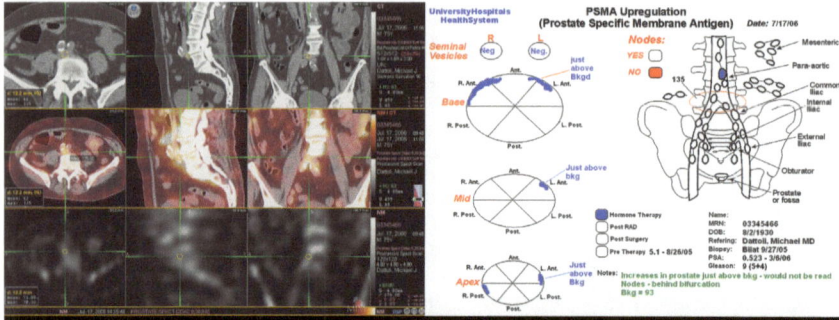

Images 11: A number of diagnostic imaging techniques for lymph node involvement can be fused with helical CT or with MRI or with CT/PET scans. A pictorial analysis for this patient appears to the right of the scanned images.

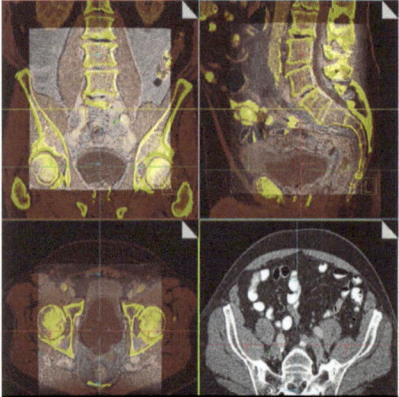

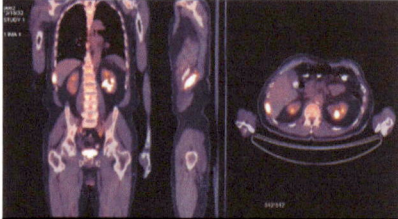

Image 12: The first three images (top right/left and bottom left) are of the abdomen and pelvis in saggital, coronal and axial views. They are MRI fused images that highlight bony anatomy and enhance organs with a rich blood supply. On the first of these images, you can see the right and left kidneys in the upper part of the frame. The last of the four images (bottom right) is a CT scan of the abdomen used to correlate with the fused MRI images for reference.

Image 13: The 18F-Fluoride PET/CT imaging technique has demonstrated 100% predictive accuracy (sensitivity and specificity), which is as good as it gets. The images show a biopsy-proven skeletal lesion (metastatic prostate cancer) in one rib, which proved to be treatable. We've pushed the envelope with respect to where we can treat, because the technologies are now so advanced.

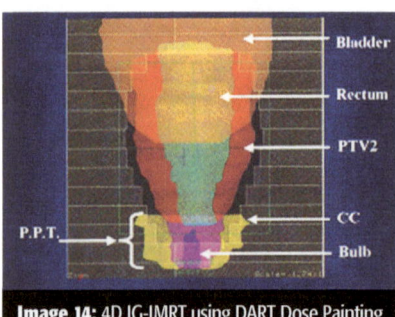

Image 14: 4D IG-IMRT using DART Dose Painting.

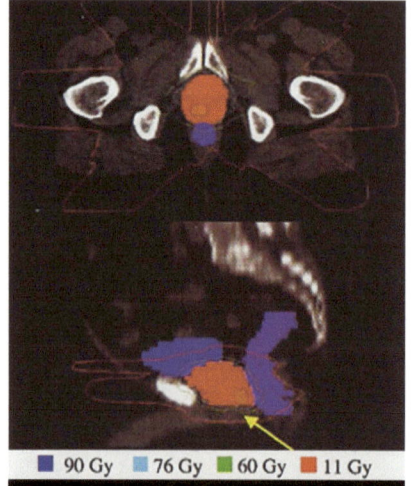

Image 15: 4D IG-IMRT Treatment Plan.

APPENDIX C

A SUMMARY OF THE 16-YEAR DATA

The following summary is based on a Dattoli series that was first presented at an American Society of Clinical Oncology meeting (February, 2009), and subsequently published in the *Journal of Oncology* (Dattoli M, Wallner K True L, Bostwick D, Cash J, Sorace, R, Long-term Outcomes for Patients with Prostate Cancer having Intermediate and High-risk Disease, treated with Brachytherapy and Supplemental External Beam Radiotherapy, J Oncol. 2010; pii: 471375. Epub 2010 Aug 18). The summary also draws on an earlier published series (Dattoli M, et al., *Urology*, 2007 Feb; 69(2):334-337).

The bottom line in our clinical studies is that these are patients who were at high risk, with a high likelihood of extraprostatic extension (cancer that has spread outside the prostate gland). These patients were first treated with 3D-Conformal Radiation Therapy—3D-CRT (which was the state-of-the-art approach prior to the more recent IMRT era) followed by brachytherapy. The study was by a single author-practitioner doing the implants, but the biochemical data was independently reviewed by the University of Washington, and all the slides were re-reviewed by the University of Washington, which adds an element of security to the data. Clinical stage was not included because the doctors at the University of Washington couldn't perform a digital rectal exam on these patients due to geographical distance. These results will serve as a baseline for comparison with the various alternative treatment options discussed in this booklet.

It should be noted that DART is far more precise and delivers a significantly higher dose than 3D-CRT. A number of studies have shown that higher doses greatly increase the likelihood of patients being cancer-free after treatment. At our center, we have been employing DART in our combined protocol with brachytherapy since 2005, and during the intervening years, we are confident that our results have further improved even since we first reported our 16-year series.

Materials and Methods
321 Consecutive Patients treated by one author (M.D.)–157 intermediate risk and 164 high risk.

Selection Criteria
NCCN Guidelines

Radiation Treatment Regimen
- 3D-CRT Dose: 4140cGy Median (Range 39 Gy–54 Gy)
- Pd-103 Dose: 8000-9000 Minimum Peripheral Dose (pre-NIST-99)
- Source Strength: 1.4 mCi Median (Range 1.1-1.6 mCi)
- Clinical Pd-103 Target Volume: extended 0.5 – 1.0 cm, antero-laterally to the TRUS prostate margin
- Patients were followed at 3, 6 and 12 months, and every 6-12 months thereafter
- Definition of biochemical success: PSA ≤ 0.2 ng/ml, nadir +2 and ASTRO Consensus Definition
- Follow-up saturation prostate biopsies were performed on all failing patients
- Biochemical data independently re-reviewed and analyzed by Kent Wallner, MD (Univ. of Washington)
- Original biopsy slides re-reviewed by Lawrence True, MD (Univ. of Washington)
- Clinical stage was not included in final data analysis to reduce subjectivity

Patient Characteristics
- Mean PSA 19.4 (1.6–147)
- Median PSA 16.4
- 218 Patients had Gleason Score 7-10
- 203 Patients had PSA > 10
- 79 Patients had elevated PAPs
- 141 Patients had Clinical Stage T2C
- 127 Patients had Clinical Stage T3

Follow-up
- 16 year actuarial, Median 10.3 years
- 143 Patients received a median of 4 months neo-adjuvant or adjuvant therapy

Results

➢ PAP was the strongest predictor of failure (p= 0.0001), followed by Gleason Score (p< 0.001) and PSA (p=0.03)

➢ Hormones conferred no survival advantage (p=0.4) although patients receiving hormones had the most adverse features

➢ 82% overall actuarial freedom from biochemical progress at 16 years using strict PSA nadir of ≤0.2 ng/ml (Freedom from failure calculated by method of Kaplan-Meier. Difference between groups were determined by the log rank or students' t-test) (86% cancer specific survival; 89% intermediate and 74% high risk)

➢ The absolute risk of failure fell to 1% beyond 5 years after treatment

➢ Treatment morbidity was limited to RTOG grade 1-2 symptoms. No patients experienced grade 3-4 toxicity. (One patient who had both a TURP and TUIP developed low-volume stress incontinence.) No patient developed rectal ulceration

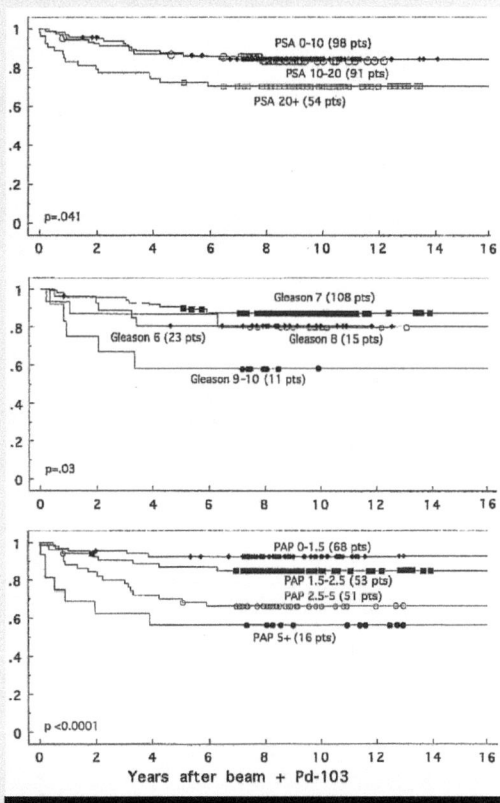

These three graphs show the freedom of biographical progression of the disease out to 16 years stratified by PSA, Gleason Score, and PAP.

➢ All failing patients underwent prostatic biopsies. There were no pathologically documented local failures

Conclusions

➢ Patients having high risk prostate cancer may enjoy long-term biochemical freedom even when using strict PSA nadirs

➢ Morbidity has been very acceptable

- Despite the aggressive nature of this study group, no local failures have been documented
- It is encouraging that the failure rate decreased to near zero with follow-up beyond 5 years
- These results appear superior to surgery, aggressive external beam radiotherapy (including full course IMRT ± hormones, protons/neutrons or combined radiation methods using other isotopes ± hormones) in this high risk group
- We attribute these exceedingly favorable results, in part, to our effort to achieve wide brachytherapy treatment margins. This is accomplished by using highly peripheral and extra-capsular source placement
- Pd-103 appears to be the isotope best suited for high-risk cancers

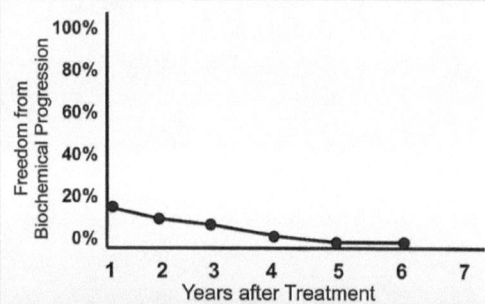

This graph shows the likelihood of subsequent bio-chemical failure versus years after treatment. These results are encouraging because as time goes on fewer and fewer patients experience biochemical failure, indicated by a PSA greater than 0.2.

NOTE: A 2017 multi-institutional study led by the UCLA Jonsson Comprehensive Cancer Center employed a combined radiation protocol similar to that utilized at our institution to treat high-risk patients. With very aggressive cancers (defined as Gleason score 9-10), the UCLA researchers reported that "extremely-dose escalated radiotherapy" combining EBRT and brachytherapy "with short-course androgen deprivation therapy offered the least risk of developing metastases" (Kishan, AU, et al, Eur Urol. 2017 May; 71(5):766-773). These results for high-risk patients treated with high dose combination radiotherapy are consistent with our own 16-year outcomes.

APPENDIX D

SURVEY COMPARING PRIMARY TREATMENT MODALITIES

In 2011, the Prostate Cancer Treatment Center of Seattle, Washington published the first of a series of retrospective studies comparing all currently available primary treatment options. This annual survey is conducted by the Prostate Cancer Results Study Group (PCRSG), an international team comprised of leading prostate cancer researchers who have exhaustively analyzed the peer-reviewed studies from 2000 to June 2017. The data for those studies was used to rigorously compare results reported for the following primary treatments:

- Surgery (Radical Prostatectomy—RP & Robotic)
- External Beam Radiation Therapy (EBRT—including IMRT)
- Brachytherapy (Seeds)
- External Beam Radiation Therapy & Brachytherapy Combined
- High Frequency Ultrasound (HIFU)
- Proton Therapy (Protons)
- Cryotherapy (Cryo)

The thousands of studies reviewed by the PCRSG team had to meet strict criteria that would qualify them for inclusion in the survey analysis, including the number of patients who were treated and the number of years of patient follow-up, with a minimum of 5 years. The definitions of biochemical disease-free survival, clinical staging and risk stratification (low, intermediate and high) were also evaluated.

Based on the reported clinical outcomes of the studies that were reviewed, the conclusions of the PCRSG team were ordered according to low, intermediate and high-risk groups. The Dattoli team contributed to the survey early on, and the most recent survey confirms the Dattoli combined protocol (EBRT and Seeds, with or without hormonal therapy) as the most effective long-term treatment for both intermediate and high-risk patients.

For high-risk patients, the PCRSG offered the following analysis. "Patients with Gleason Scores 8-10, Stage T2c or T3, A PSA greater than 20, or two intermediate factors, such as a PSA 10-20 and Gleason Score 7, are considered to have high risk disease. High risk simply means that there is a higher risk that disease is outside the prostate.

"Estimates of risk of disease beyond the prostate range from 23-88%. Most patients in this group have a risk of at least 50%, making them poor candidates for treatments that treat the prostate alone (i.e. surgery, seed implantation alone, EBRT to just the prostate)." The results for surgery, for example, demonstrate that only 25-50% of patients will be successfully treated with radical prostatectomy.

"The triple modality approach (External Beam, Seed Implantation and Hormonal Therapy) for High Risk disease begins with the rationale that Hormonal Therapy may reduce the number of cells that need to be killed. EBRT (IMRT) can deliver an adequate dose to kill microscopic disease beyond the gland and seed implantation can deliver a dose sufficient to control the disease within the gland."

With regard to the combined protocol, the PCRSG team concluded, "this rationale may be supported with cancer control rates long term of 85-92%." Those results are consistent with those reported by the Dattoli team and are dramatically superior to the clinical outcomes reported with other treatment modalities, as illustrated in the following PCRSG graphs for intermediate and high risk patients. Results similar to our combined radiotherapy protocol for high risk patients (Gleason score 9-10) were also reported by researchers at UCLA (Kishan AU, et al, Eur Urol, 2017 May;71(5):766-773).

CLOSING NOTE

While this booklet seeks to provide the reader with a complete review of current prostate cancer treatments it will do you well to understand that a highly competitive market for patients provides fertile ground for "creative marketing." Many treatment facilities are actively advertising their services using fabricated words or quasi trademarks to attempt to set themselves apart from the rest. There is a "new – latest – best" creation nearly every month. We encourage you to look *beyond* the marketing hype to the true essence of the physician's practice: how long has he/she been performing the procedure they recommend? How many patients with similar disease characteristics like yours has he/she treated? What was the documented success? Does the physician or practice have long-term results and are they published in a peer-reviewed medical journal? And if the physician is suggesting a treatment that he or she does not do personally (for example, a Urologist sending you to a radiation center), you would be wise to ask if you are being referred to a facility in which your physician has a financial interest.

APPENDIX E

DECIDING WHAT IS BEST FOR YOU

Consult with your physician, and by all means, obtain second and third opinions whenever possible, preferably from physicians with different specialties. If you have already been to a urologist, it is worthwhile to visit a radiation oncologist or medical oncologist (those with experience with hormones and chemotherapy).

Join a support group such as US TOO!, or PAACT. If you belong to any of the computer on-line services, check out the medical and health bulletin boards and mailing lists for the latest information and announcements for prostate cancer patients. Keep your personal plan of action updated.

What to Remember

- Obtain all of the advice and counsel that you can, but keep in mind that the decisions are ultimately yours to make.

- Be positive—if you have been properly staged and treated, the odds are in your favor on not having a recurrence.

- If you should have a rising PSA over time after initial treatment, don't panic. Get further tests, and if appropriate, get a biopsy, preferably guided by Color-Flow Power Doppler Ultrasound.

- The secret to success with prostate cancer is catching the disease early, and that is also true for recurrence.

- If testing confirms cancer, learn all you can about your options. Get second and third opinions. Become informed and empowered. Become involved with solving your problem. It's your life and body. Go for it!

- Life is full of problems and challenges. Solve this problem like any other big problem:
    1. Identify the problem.
    2. Get all the facts to confirm that you have a problem.
    3. Learn what options are available to you and weigh them carefully.
    4. Choose a qualified doctor who is experienced and with whom you are comfortable.
    5. Initiate and follow through with the solution.
- Don't be afraid to ask for help from your spouse or partner, from your family and your friends. It is more important than ever for you to turn to loved ones to get the emotional and spiritual support you need. This disease can be a difficult struggle for us, but we are not alone, and our mental attitude, prayers and our fighting spirit really can make all the difference.

To be a cancer survivor, you must first be a cancer fighter!

APPENDIX F

GLOSSARY OF MEDICAL TERMS

3D-CRT (3-Dimensional Conformal Radiation Therapy): See Conformal Radiotherapy.

5-alpha reductase (5-AR): an enzyme that converts testosterone to dihydrotestosterone (DHT).

Adenocarcinoma: A cancer originating in glandular tissue. Prostate cancer is classified as adenocarcinoma of the prostate.

Adjuvant: An additional treatment used to increase the effectiveness of the primary therapy. Radiation therapy and hormonal therapy are often used as adjuvant treatments following a radical prostatectomy. Compare Neoadjuvant.

Agonist: A chemical substance that combines with a receptor on a cell and initiates an activity or reaction. See LHRH analogs.

Algorithm: A step-by-step procedure for solving a problem or accomplishing some end, especially by a computer.

Analog: A man-made chemical compound that is structurally similar to one produced naturally by the body. See LHRH analogs.

Anastomotic stricture: narrowing, usually by scarring, of an anastomotic suture line.

Androgen: A hormone that produces male characteristics. See testosterone.

Androgen ablation therapy: A therapy designed to inhibit the body's production of testosterones.

Androgen-dependent cells: Prostate cancer cells which are nourished by male hormones and therefore are capable of being destroyed by hormone deprivation (also known as androgen-sensitive cells).

Androgen-independent cells: Prostate cancer cells which are not dependent on male hormones and therefore do not respond to hormonal therapy (also known as androgen-insensitive cells).

Anesthetic: A drug that produces general or local loss of physical sensations, particularly pain. A "spinal" is the injection of a local anesthetic into the area surrounding the spinal cord.

Aneuploid: Having an abnormal number of chromosomes, as revealed by ploidy analysis. Aneuploid prostate cancer cells tend not to respond well to androgen deprivation therapy (ADT).

Angiogenesis: The body's formation of new blood vessels. Some anti-cancer drugs work by blocking angiogenesis, thus preventing blood from reaching and nourishing a tumor.

Antagonist: A chemical substance in the body that acts to reduce the physiological activity of another chemical substance.

Antiandrogens: Drugs such as Casodex that block the activity of androgens produced by the adrenal glands at the cellular receptor sites. Androgens can block or neutralize the effects of testosterone and DHT on prostate cancer cells.

Antibody: A protein produced by the body that counteracts the toxic effects of a foreign substance, organism, or disease within the body.

Antigen: A foreign substance such as a virus or bacterium that causes an immune response or the formation of an antibody.

Antineoplastic: Inhibits growth and proliferation of cancer cells.

Antioxidants: Any substances which delay the process of oxidation in the body.

Apoptosis: The normal molecular mechanism which governs the life span of cells so that they die in a very organized way. Cancerous cells are resistant to normal apoptosis.

Benign: A non-cancerous condition. See also Benign Prostatic Hypertrophy.

Benign Prostatic Hypertrophy (BPH): Also called Benign Prostatic Hyperplasia, BPH is a non-cancerous condition of the prostate that results in a growth of tumorous tissue and increase in the size of the prostate.

Biopsy: A procedure involving the removal of tissue from the body of the patient. Removed tissue is typically examined microscopically by a pathologist in order to make a precise diagnosis of the patient's condition.

Bone scan: An imaging technique used to detect bone metastases, which appear as "hot spots" on the film. It is far more sensitive than the conventional x-ray.

BPH: See Benign Prostatic Hypertrophy.

Brachytherapy: A form of radiation therapy in which radioactive seeds are implanted into the prostate to deliver radiation directly to the tumor. Also referred to as seed implantation, or seeding.

Cancer: A cellular malignancy typically forming tumors. Unlike benign tumors, these tend to invade surrounding tissues and spread to distant sites of the body.

Carcinoma: A malignant tumor made up chiefly of epithelial cells, or those cells that form the lining of an organ or cavity. See Adenocarcinoma.

Castrate Range: The level of the body's testosterone after orchiectomy (also referred to as castration). This is the range or level, which is used by physicians as a point of comparison for those drugs, which attempt to decrease the testosterone level.

CAT Scan (or CT Scan): See Computer Tomography.

cGy: Abbreviation for centigray; a unit of radiation equivalent to the older unit called a "rad."

Chemotherapy: The treatment of cancer using chemicals that deter the growth of cancer cells.

Collimator: A device that organizes radiation such that only parallel rays or beams emanate.

Combination Hormonal Therapy (CHT): Also referred to as Combined Hormonal Blockade (CHB), or Combined Androgen Deprivation Therapy (ADT). The preferred term is ADT, often designated with a number referring to the number of agents used (i.e., monotherapy ADT, ADT2, ADT3). This combined therapy can utilize a number of mechanisms, including surgical or medical ADT, antiandrogens, 5-alpha reductase inhibitors, estrogenic compounds, agents that block adrenal androgen production, and agents that decrease the receptivity of the androgen receptor.

Combination Therapy: Refers generally to any combination of treatment modalities used to treat prostate cancer.

Computer Tomography: Computer generated cross-sectional images of a portion of the body. Also called CT or CAT scan.

Conformal Radiotherapy: A radiation treatment conforming precisely to the size and shape of the prostate, with the use of computerized planning and state-of-the-art imaging techniques. 3-Dimensional Conformal Radiation Therapy (3D-CRT) utilizes this sophisticated approach to treatment planning, as does the even more advanced Intensity Modulated Radiation Therapy (IMRT).

Cryosurgery (also referred to as Cryotherapy or Cryoablation): The freezing of tissue with the use of liquid nitrogen or Argon gas probes. When used to treat prostate cancer, the cryoprobes are guided by transrectal ultrasound.

Cytokine: Any of a class of immunoregulatory substances that are secreted by cells of the immune system.

DHT (dihydrotestosterone): The active form of the male hormone, testosterone, produced after testosterone is transformed by an enzyme known as 5-alpha reductase.

Diagnosis: Evaluation of a patient's symptoms and/or test results, with the intent of identifying and verifying the existence of any underlying disease or abnormal condition.

Digital Rectal Examination (DRE): A procedure in which the physician inserts a gloved, lubricated finger into the rectum to examine the prostate gland for signs of cancer.

DNA (Deoxyribonucleic Acid): A complex protein that is the carrier of genetic information that determines the physical development and growth of living organisms.

Doppler Ultrasound Technique: A machine that sends out ultrasonic waves that pick up the velocity of blood flow through the veins and are transmitted as sound to make an image.

Doubling Time: The time it takes for a tumor or cancerous focus to double in size.

Downsizing: The use of hormonal therapy or other forms of intervention to reduce tumor volume prior to primary, curative treatment.

Downstaging: The use of hormonal therapy or other forms of intervention to lower the clinical stage of prostate cancer prior to primary, curative treatment.

Ejaculatory Ducts: The tubular passages through which semen reaches the prostatic urethra during orgasm.

Ejaculation: The release of semen through the penis during orgasm.

Endorectal MRI: Magnetic resonance imaging of the prostate gland using a probe inserted into the rectum. Dynamic Contrast Enhanced MRI is the most effective form of magnetic resonance imaging.

Enzyme: A chemical substance produced by living cells that causes chemical reactions to take place while not being changed itself.

Erectile Dysfunction (also referred to as ED or impotence): The loss of ability to produce and/or sustain an erection sufficient for intercourse.

Estrogen: A female sex hormone that can be used as a form of therapy to inhibit the production of testosterone in patients diagnosed with prostate cancer.

External Beam Radiation Therapy (EBRT): A form of radiation therapy that utilizes radiation delivered by an external source (machine) and directed at a target area to be radiated. In contrast to EBRT, brachytherapy utilizes radiation sources (seeds) that are internal, implanted in the target tissue. EBRT may use conventional photons, protons, neutrons or electrons.

Extraprostatic Extension: Used to describe prostate cancer that has spread outside the prostate gland.

False Negative: An erroneous negative test result. For example, an imaging test that fails to show the presence of a cancer tumor later found by biopsy to be present in the patient is said to have returned a false negative result.

False Positive: A positive test result that mistakenly identifies a state or condition that does not in fact exist.

Feraheme (Ferumoxytol): A ferromagnetic nanoparticle which is taken up by normal macrophages with the lymph nodes.

Fistula: With regard to prostate cancer, an abnormal passage due to injury or disease that connects an abscess or hollow organ to the surface of the body or to another hollow organ. If there is significant damage to the rectal wall proximate to the bladder, a fistula may occur between the bladder and rectum.

Flare Reaction: A testosterone surge caused by the initial use of an LHRH analog, causing a temporary increase of tumor growth and symptoms (known as clinical flare), or an increase in PSA (biochemical flare).

Foley Catheter: A catheter inserted in the penis and threaded through the urethra to the bladder where it is held in place with a tiny, inflated balloon. It removes urine from the bladder and can be used to irrigate the urethra and prevent blood clots.

Free PSA: PSA that is unattached to any major protein in the blood. Free PSA is associated with benign prostate growth. The percentage of free PSA is derived by dividing the free-PSA level by the total-PSA x 100. Studies have show that men with free PSA % > 25% were at low risk for prostate cancer, while men with PSA % < 10% were at high risk for having prostate cancer.

Frozen Section: A technique in which removed tissue is frozen, cut into thin slices, and stained for microscopic examination. A pathologist can rapidly complete a frozen section analysis, and for this reason, it is commonly used during surgery to quickly provide the surgeon with vital information.

Gland: An aggregation of cells (a structure or organ) that secretes a substance for use or discharge from the body.

Gland Volume: The size in cubic centimeters (cc) or grams of the prostate gland.

Gleason Score: A widely used method for classifying the cellular differentiation of cancerous tissue. The less the cancerous cells appear like normal cells, the more malignant the cancer. Two grades of 1-5, identifying the two most common degrees of differentiation present in the examined tissue sample, are added together to produce the Gleason score. High numbers indicate greater differentiation and more aggressive cancer. The grading system is named after its originator, Donald Gleason, M.D.

Globulin: Any of a number of simple proteins that occur widely in plant and animal tissues.

Gynecomastia: A side effect involving breast enlargement and tenderness, associated with various hormonal therapies that increase the level of estrogens in the body.

HDR brachytherapy: High Dose Rate brachytherapy involves the temporary insertion of radioactive iridium isotopes into the prostate gland using transrectal ultrasound guidance.

Hematuria: Blood in the urine.

Hereditary: Inherited genetically from parents and earlier generations.

Holistic Medicine: Medical care, which considers the patient as a whole, including his or her physical, mental, emotional, spiritual, social and economic needs.

Hormone: A substance produced by one tissue or gland and transported by the bloodstream to another to effect or regulate physiological activity such as metabolism and growth.

Hormonal therapy: Cancer treatment involving the blockage of hormone production by surgical or chemical means. Because prostate cancer is usually dependent on male hormones to grow, hormonal therapy can be an effective means of alleviating symptoms and retarding the development of the disease.

Hormone refractory prostate cancer: Prostate cancer that is androgen independent, and therefore, unresponsive to hormonal therapies.

Hot Flash: A side effect of some forms of hormonal therapy, experienced as a sudden rush of warmth to the face, neck, and upper body.

Imaging: Radiology techniques that are often computer-enhanced and allow the physician to visualize areas inside the body that would not normally be visible.

Impotence: See Erectile Dysfunction.

Incontinence: A loss of urinary control. There are various kinds and degrees of incontinence. Overflow incontinence is a condition in which the bladder retains urine after voiding. As a consequence, the bladder remains full most of the time, resulting in involuntary seepage of urine from the bladder. Stress incontinence is the involuntary discharge of urine when there is increased pressure upon the bladder, as in coughing or straining to lift heavy objects. Total incontinence is the failure of ability to voluntarily exercise control over the sphincters of the bladder neck and urethra, resulting in total loss of retentive ability.

Inflammation: Redness or swelling caused by injury or infection.

Informed Consent: Permission to proceed given by a patient after being fully informed of the purposes and potential consequences of a medical procedure.

Intensity Modulated Radiation Therapy (IMRT): The most recent state-of-the-art, computer-aided technique for delivering higher doses of radiation more accurately than either conventional External Beam Radiation or Conformal Radiation. The most advanced form of IMRT is Dynamic Adaptive Radiotherapy (DART).

Intermittent Androgen Deprivation (IAD): A temporary discontinuation of hormonal therapy that allows for a return to natural testosterone production in order to spare the patient from symptoms associated with androgen deprivation. Also referred to as Intermittent Hormonal Therapy (IHT).

Intravenous Pyelogram (IVP): A test that utilizes the injection of a special dye to check for injury or the spread of cancer to the kidneys and bladder.

Investigational: A drug or procedure allowed by the FDA for use in clinical trails, but not necessarily reimbursed.

Isodose Line: A line or two-dimensional shape that circumscribes an area receiving a radiation dose greater than or equal to a specified amount.

Laparoscopic Lymphadenectomy: The removal of pelvic lymph nodes with a laparoscope via four small incisions in the lower abdomen.

LH (Luteinizing Hormone): A chemical signal originating in the pituitary gland that causes the testes to make testosterone.

LHRH Analogs (or LHRH Agonists): Synthetic compounds that are chemically similar to Luteinizing Hormone Releasing Hormone (LHRH), used to suppress testicular production of testosterone. The most commonly prescribed LHRH analogs are Lupron® and Zoldex® Eligard® and Trelstar®. See also Luteinizing Hormone-Releasing Hormone (LHRH).

LHRH Antagonist: A chemical agent that blocks the LHRH receptor without the testosterone surge associated with

LHRH analogs. LHRH antagonists include Abarelix (Plenaxis®).

Linear Accelerator: A high energy x-ray machine generating radiation fields for external beam radiation therapy. These machines are typically mounted with a collimator (or multileaf collimator) in a gantry that rotates vertically around the patient being treated.

Localized Prostate Cancer: Cancer that is confined to the prostate gland, and therefore, considered curable.

Luteinizing Hormone-Releasing Hormone (LHRH): A chemical signal originating in the hypothalamus that causes the pituitary to make LH, which in turn stimulates the testicles to make testosterone.

Lymphadenectomy: The removal and examination of lymph nodes to precisely diagnose and stage cancer. See also Laparascopic Lymphadenectomy.

Lymph Node: A small, bean-shaped mass of tissue located throughout the body along the vessels of the lymphatic system. The lymph nodes filter out bacteria and other toxins, as well as cancer cells.

Magnetic Resonance Imaging (MRI): A painless, non-invasive technique using strong magnetic fields to produce detailed images of internal body structures. An MRI scan usually takes about 45 minutes per site.

Malignancy: A tumorous growth of cancer cells.

Malignant: Having the invasive and metastatic properties of cancer. Tending to become progressively worse and to result in death.

Margin: See Surgical Margin.

Metalloprotease Inhibitors: Drugs used to suppress the body's production of certain enzymes.

Metastasis: The spread of cancer, by way of the blood stream or lymphatic system, beyond the boundaries of the organ or structure where the cancer originated. Metastases is the plural. Metastatic refers to the characteristics associated with cancer that has spread or a secondary tumor.

Metastatic Work-Up: A group of tests, including bone scans, x-rays, and blood tests, to ascertain whether cancer has metastasized.

Monoclonal Antibody (mAb): An antibody that is directed against one specific protein (antigen).

Morbidity: Unhealthy consequences and complications resulting from treatment.

MRI: See Magnetic Resonance Imaging.

Nadir: The lowest point. Doctors sometimes use this as a verb to describe return of cancer or treatment failure. The PSA nadir refers to a minimum PSA value that should be maintained after treatment if the cancer has been successfully eradicated.

Necrosis: Death of cells or tissues caused by disease or injury.

Neoadjuvant: The use of a different type of therapy before primary, curative treatment. For example, neoadjuvant Androgen Deprivation Therapy is often used prior to radiation therapy or radical surgery, with the intent of improving the effectiveness of the primary treatment by reducing the size of the tumor and/or prostate gland.

Nerve-sparing: A procedure used during radical prostatectomy in which the surgeon attempts to save the nerves (neurovascular bundles) that allow for normal sexual functions.

Neurovascular Bundles: Strands of interwoven nerves and veins that run down the side of the prostate. The bundles contain microscopic nerves that are essential for erection; they also contain arteries and veins. Cutting the nerves in the bundles during surgery, or otherwise harming them in another procedure, usually renders the patient impotent.

Nocturia: Getting up at night to urinate.

Non-invasive: Not involving any incision in the body.

Oncogenes: Genes associated with tumor growth.

Oncology: The branch of medical science dealing with tumors. A medical oncologist is a specialist in the study of cancerous tumors.

Organ-confined Disease (OCD): Prostate cancer that is confined to the prostate gland, as indicated clinically or pathologically.

Orchiectomy: A simple operation that involves surgical removal of the testicles, which produce most of the body's testosterone.

Osteoporosis: A decrease in bone mass and density causing fragility and porosity.

Overstaging: An assessment of an overly high clinical stage at initial diagnosis.

Palliative: Affording symptomatic pain relieve but not cure or remission.

Palpable: Capable of being felt when examined by touch or manipulation.

PAP: See Prostatic Acid Phosphatase.

Pathologist: A doctor who specializes in the examination of cells and tissues removed from the body.

PBRT: See Proton Beam Radiation Therapy.

Perineum: The area of the body between the anus and scrotum. A perineal procedure uses this area as the point of entry into the body.

Perineural Invasion: Describing cancer, which has spread from the prostate to the nerve bundles.

Periprostatic: Relating to the soft tissues immediately proximate to the prostate gland.

Photon: The quantum of electromagnetic energy, described as having zero mass and no electric charge. X-rays are high energy photons.

Placebo: A sugar pill often taken by participants in a medical study. Patients taking a placebo are compared to patients taking actual medications.

Ploidy Analysis: A pathological analysis to determine the number of sets of chromosomes in a cell.

Proctitis: Inflammation of the rectum.

Prognosis: A forecast of the course of a disease and future prospects of the patient.

Progression: A change in the status of the cancer indicating the condition has progressed and worsened.

Pro-oxidant: A term to describe substances that aid in oxidation.

ProstaScint® Scan: An imaging technique sometimes used determine whether or not cancer has spread to distant sites by using monoclonal antibodies.

Prostate Capsule: It was once thought that the prostate gland was surrounded by a clearly identifiable capsule, but pathological studies have shown there is no capsule as such. The gland exists within a fat plane.

Prostatectomy: The surgical removal of part or all of the prostate gland.

Prostate Specific Antigen (PSA): A blood test that measures a substance manufactured solely by prostate gland cells. An elevated reading indicates an abnormal condition of the prostate gland, either benign or malignant. It is presently the most sensitive tumor marker for the identification and monitoring of prostate cancer.

Prostatic Acid Phosphatase (PAP): An enzyme produced by the prostate that is elevated (3.0 or higher) in many patients when prostate cancer has spread beyond the prostate.

Prostatitis: An infection or inflammation of the prostate gland that is treatable with medications.

Proton Beam Radiation Therapy (PBRT): A form of radiation therapy that utilizes protons as the source of energy (as opposed to X-rays or neutrons).

PSA: See Prostate Specific Antigen.

PSA Bounce (or PSA Bump): A rise in PSA level after first having a reduction in PSA after radiation therapy.

PSA Nadir: The lowest PSA value after a particular treatment.

PSA Velocity (PSAV): The rate of increase of the PSA level, expressed as nanograms per milliliter per year.

Radiation Therapy (RT): The use of high energy rays to kill cancer cells and malignant tissue.

Radiation Urethritis: Inflammation of the urethra caused by radiation therapy.

Radical Prostatectomy: An operation to remove the entire prostate gland and seminal vesicles.

Radiosensitivity: The degree to which a type of cancer responds to radiation therapy.

RBA or Relative Biological Effectiveness: A scale used to compare the intensity of radiation associated with various atomic particles.

Receptor: A cellular docking site that interacts with a specific protein or enzyme (called a ligand). The interaction typically leads to the synthesis of other substances such as proteins, hormones or enzymes.

Recurrence: Return of the cancer following remission or treatment intended as curative. Local recurrence indicates a return of the cancer at the site of origin. Distant recurrence indicates the appearance of one or more metastases of the disease.

Refractory: A term indicating that the cancer no longer responds to the current therapy.

Remission: Complete or partial disappearance of the signs and symptoms of the disease. The period during which a disease remains under control, without progressing. Even complete remission does not necessarily indicate cure.

Resection: The surgical removal of a part of an organ or structure.

Risk: The probability that a particular event will or will not happen.

RP: See Radical Prostatectomy.

RT: See Radiation Therapy.

Rx: The standard abbreviation for prescription.

Salvage Treatment: A medical term for "Plan B." It means a patient must undergo another form of treatment because the first therapy was not successful. Salvage therapy may incur a higher rate of side effects.

Saw Palmetto: A nutrient extracted from the saw palmetto shrub, which is considered by some to aid the body's immune system.

Seed Implantation (SI): A minimally invasive procedure by which radioactive seeds are implanted into the prostate gland to destroy cancer. Also referred to as seeding and brachytherapy.

Selenium: A non-metallic element thought to be beneficial as a nutrient; it is often included in multivitamin supplements.

Seminal Vesicles: Glands that, like the prostate, support male reproduction. Fluid secreted by these glands regulates the consistency of semen.

Side Effect: A reaction to a treatment or medication, usually referring to an undesirable effect.

Sphincter: A circular muscle which contracts to close an orifice. The urethral sphincter squeezes the urethra shut, providing urinary control.

Staging: The testing process by which the extent and severity of a known cancer is evaluated according to an established system of classification. It is used to help determine appropriate therapy. See TNM Staging and Whitmore-Jewett Staging.

Surgical Margin: The outer edge of the tissue removed during a radical prostatectomy. The surgical margin may be "negative," indicating that no cancer is present and a better prognosis, or "positive," indicating that not all of the cancer has been removed.

Systemic: Throughout the body and affecting the entire body.

T-Cell: An immune system cell or lymphocyte that directs an immune response to malignant or infected cells.

Testes: Two male reproductive glands located inside the scrotum. The testes are the primary sources for testosterone. Also called testicles.

Testosterone: A male sex hormone chiefly produced by the testicles.

Thrombotic: Causing or relating to blood clotting.

TNM Staging: The most widely used classification system for evaluating the extent of prostate cancer. TNM refers to tumor, nodes and metastases. See Staging.

Transrectal: Through the rectum.

Transurethral: Through the urethra.

Transrectal Ultrasonography: See Ultrasound.

Transurethral Resection of the Prostate (TURP): A surgical procedure to remove tissue obstructing the urethra. The technique involves the insertion of an instrument called a resectoscope into the penile urethra, and is intended to relieve obstruction of urine flow due to enlargement of the prostate.

Tumor: An excessive growth of cells that is caused by uncontrolled and disorderly cell replacement. Abnormal tissue growth may be benign or malignant. See also Benign, Malignant.

TURP: See Transurethral Resection of the Prostate.

Ultrasound (Transrectal Ultrasonography): A painless, non-invasive diagnostic imaging technique using sound waves to create an echo pattern that reveals the structure of organs and tissues. It does not use x-rays.

Understaging: An overly low assessment of clinical stage at diagnosis.

Urethra: The tube that carries urine from the bladder and semen from the prostate out of the body through the penis.

Urologist: A physician who specializes in the diagnosis and the medical and surgical treatment of problems in the urinary and male reproductive systems.

USPIO: This technology uses ultrasmall superparamagnetic iron oxide (USPIO) as an MRI contrast agent for the identification of cancer metastasis in lymph nodes.

Vasectomy: A surgical procedure to render a man sterile by cutting the vas deferens, thus eliminating the passage of sperm from the testes to the prostate.

Vasoactive: Causing the dilation or constriction of blood vessels.

Vesicle: A small sac containing fluid, as in seminal vesicles.

Whitmore-Jewett Staging: A classification system for evaluating the extent of prostate cancer. This system is less widely used for the designation of stage than is TNM staging.

X-rays: High energy radiation that can be used at low levels of intensity to make images of the body's internal structures, or at high intensity for radiation therapy.

APPENDIX G

THE WARNING SIGNS OF PROSTATE CANCER

There are often no warning signs of prostate cancer. In some cases the following symptoms may indicate the presence of the disease. However, please be aware that these symptoms may also be due to benign conditions of the prostate, or other conditions entirely unrelated to prostate cancer:

- ✓ Elevated or rising PSA
- ✓ Abnormal Digital Rectal Exam
- ✓ Blood in urine
- ✓ Pain or difficulty urinating
- ✓ Increased urge to urinate, especially at night
- ✓ Hesitant or intermittent urinary flow
- ✓ Pain or discomfort in area of prostate
- ✓ Unusual and unexplained weight loss
- ✓ Continual pain in lower back, hips or pelvis
- ✓ Increased voiding urgency
- ✓ Inability to urinate
- ✓ Trouble having or keeping an erection (erectile dysfunction)
- ✓ Weakness or numbness in the legs or feet

ABOUT THE AUTHOR

Michael J. Dattoli, MD

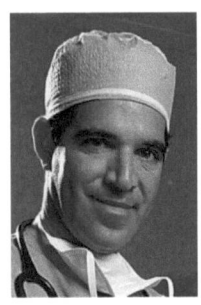

Michael J. Dattoli, MD, is a board-certified radiation oncologist with well over two decades of brachytherapy experience and has performed thousands of prostate implant procedures. He is considered the foremost pioneer in the field, optimizing brachytherapy designs to maximize tumor eradication and minimize symptoms. He has also been the leading trailblazer in the development of Dynamic Adaptive Radiotherapy (DART), utilizing all of the state-of-the-art modalities associated with 4-Dimensional Image-Guided Intensity Modulated Radiotherapy (3D-IMRT). Dr. Dattoli has successfully applied the same technologies to other forms of cancer, including breast, head and neck, GI, GYN, sarcomas and lung malignancies. He is a noted author and speaker in this complex field of medicine.

Dr. Dattoli attended the University of California at Berkeley and was the Valedictorian of his class at Vassar College; he earned his medical degree at Mount Sinai School of Medicine, Radiation Oncology at New York University Medical Center, then distinguished himself at Memorial Sloan-Kettering Cancer Center and New York Hospital-Cornell University Medical Center, as the Special Fellow in Brachytherapy. He was appointed Associate Professor in Brachytherapy and Radiation Oncology at Memorial Sloan- Kettering Cancer Center in New York and at New York Hospital-Cornell University Medical Center prior to relocating to Florida.

Dr. Dattoli also serves on multiple journal editorial review boards. Government appointments include "The Prostate Cancer Task Force" in Florida and consultant to the "Washington Oncology Roundtable Advisory Committee". He was selected by the International Association of Oncologists as a Leading Physician of the World and top Brachytherapist.

THE DATTOLI CANCER FOUNDATION MISSION

The Dattoli Cancer Foundation, sponsor of the Prostate Cancer Resource Network, is a 501(c)(3), tax-exempt charitable organization, whose mission is

- to raise awareness of the wide-spread incidence of Prostate Cancer and the need for early and annual screenings;

- to provide information and support to men newly diagnosed with Prostate Cancer as well as to those with recurrent Prostate Cancer, and

- to foster research into better diagnostic tools and treatment options for Prostate Cancer.

Gifts to the Dattoli Foundation make possible publications like this one, and are welcomed anytime. A copy of the official registration and financial information may be obtained from the Division of Consumer Services by calling toll-free (800-435-7352) within the state. Registration does not imply endorsement, approval or recommendations by the state.

Dattoli Cancer Foundation
2803 Fruitville Road
Sarasota, FL 34237
941/365-5599
800/915-1001
fax: 941/330-2317
www.dattolifoundation.org

ORDER MORE BOOKLETS IN THE SERIES

This *Prostate Cancer Essentials for Survival* booklet was published by the Dattoli Cancer Foundation. For a complete list of booklets in the series and ordering information, please visit the Dattoli Cancer Center Book Shelf at dattoli.com/book-shelf. Current titles include:

- ✔ Dynamic Adaptive Radiation Therapy for Prostate Cancer
- ✔ The Dattoli Prostate Cancer Challenge: Evaluating All Your Treatment Options
- ✔ The Facts: Comparing Prostate Cancer Treatment Options
- ✔ Interpreting Your PSA Results and Related Prostate Cancer Lab Tests
- ✔ Coping with Prostate Cancer Recurrence: Advanced Diagnostics and Treatment Options
- ✔ Image-Guided Prostate Biopsy: When, Why and What to Expect
- ✔ Dosimetry and Prostate Cancer Radiotherapy
- ✔ Advanced Imaging for Prostate Cancer: A Primer on 3D Color-Flow Power Doppler Ultrasound, Multiparametric MRI and CT Fusion Techniques
- ✔ Radiation Safety and Prostate Cancer: Need You Be Concerned?
- ✔ Hormonal Therapy for Prostate Cancer: The Benefits and Risks
- ✔ Lymph Node Positive Prostate Cancer: Advanced Diagnostics and Treatment
- ✔ The Dattoli Blue Ribbon Prostate Cancer Solution: How to Survive and Thrive Without Surgery

www.ingramcontent.com/pod-product-compliance
Lightning Source LLC
Chambersburg PA
CBHW040220220526
45473CB00001B/62